Gut Check –
What's Best for Your
Digestive System

*Plus ... Inspiring Gluten Free Recipes for
Eating Healthy*

Vivianne Rankin

ISBN: 978-1952263323

Acknowledgment

I would like to acknowledge all the people who supported me throughout this book and those who evaluated every aspect of it. Those who believed in me. It is because of their constant support and trust that I was able to break through and achieve this milestone.

For Annie and Doug, the two loves of my life.

My heart truly belongs to you.

Thank you.

About the Author

Passionate about health and nutrition, and helping her clients achieve their health goals, Vivianne Rankin's philosophy centers on lifelong learning as she continues to work towards enhancing the well-being of her clients by empowering them with the knowledge, skills, support, guidance, and resources to assist and inspire them on their way to healthy living.

Vivianne stepped foot in the kitchen at the age of 9, and had since then been experimenting with homemade potato chips, cakes and creating a host of meals for her family of six. After a family member was diagnosed with a health issue, she began her research in healthy food in 2007. In 2016, Vivianne became a certified Nutritional Therapist and later, in 2018, she gained certification as a Personal Trainer.

In 2019, cancer completely changed Vivianne's life and her views about healthy living and healthy eating. This book is a glimpse of her journey towards the road of recovery and mastering the art of culinary, that she would like you to be a part of.

Preface

For most of my life I've been enjoying the process of playing with spices and unique flavors – something I've been doing since the age of 9. Growing up, I never imagined I would pursue my passion as my profession, but life had different plans for me.

After a family member was diagnosed with a critical condition, my research about food as medicine began. My work motivated me to know not just about the food I am putting on the table, but also the science behind it. I wanted to present my family with the best food, to ensure their health, fitness, and wellness.

With time, my knowledge evolved to new heights, yet my vision remained the same. Now, my efforts are not directed just towards my family, but also towards my clients.

The idea behind healthy eating is to find a regime, stick to it, and ensure that it is the best fit according to each individual's needs. Depending on your food sensitivity or allergy, you can choose a diet that best suits your body and palate.

There are so many diet choices today. The common ground between all these diet approaches is the fact that they are developed on a one size that fits all approaches. It's important to strive to cut down the unhealthy components of today's foods – GMOs, factory-farmed animals, and processed and non-organic foods – while incorporating the components of healthy food, such as wholesome fresh produce, grass-fed meat, and organically grown produce. Sticking to a natural way of living and eating foods that are as unique as you are.

In a nutshell, you have to be cognizant of all the foods that you consume because your gut is ultimately responsible for your health. Your gut health, if gone bad, can impose a major threat to your health. This is going to form the basis of the book in which we will take a detailed look at the healthy foods and healthy living.

You might choose a diet that suits your sensitivities and allergies, according to what you think your body needs. However, it needs to be kept in mind that whatever diet you choose has to as unique as you are. Gut health is essential in promoting a healthy lifestyle. A combination of lean protein along with plenty of plant based foods keeps the gut healthy.

Unfortunately, the promotion of a healthy gut is not a one size fits all program. One source of lean meat may be beneficial for one person but might not work on your neighbor. Throughout this book, I want you to be aware of the benefits of healthy eating and its impact on your life. The advantages are profound, you just need to be ready to make the most of them.

Contents

Page Left Blank Intentionally

Chapter 1
Food for Thought-
The Evolution

Like all living things, we need nutrition to survive. Looking back at how our ancestors used to eat, and comparing it to our eating habits and lifestyle of today, makes us realize how far we have come and how much our needs and wants have changed. Today, many of us are confused about what to eat and which diet to follow, what foods to eat and our overall concern about healthy eating.

With the variety of diets and nutritional approaches that have become popular over the years, it becomes increasingly difficult for an individual to stick to a single diet plan that fits his or her body requirements, and after all, there really is no 'one size fits all' meal plan. Our evolution of food consumption from ancient times, to the modern era when our palates are ruled by the immediate gratification of fast food and quick meals has taken its toll on our bodies as well as our brains.

The Food Story

As we all know, our hunter-gatherer ancestors relied solely on game and other unprocessed foods that they gathered through hunting. It's not hard to understand that the food we eat today is much different, in both nutritional content and variety than what our ancestors used to eat.

They were leaner, more muscular, and healthier. They didn't suffer from today's medical conditions, many of which have recently seen a rise– atherosclerosis, hypertension and cardiovascular disease to name a few. Many of these diseases have seen an increase as a result of consuming heavily processed foods and foods that have been exposed to extensive pesticide use.

In the span of just 23 years from 1990 to 2013, there was a 41% increase in the number of deaths resulting from cardiovascular diseases, globally.

Here's how food and nutrition have evolved from a period of raw eating, hunting, and gathering to today's large scale food production and processing.

Dairy, Poultry, and Meat

Many of our more recent ancestors grew their own vegetables and raised their own animals. Animals were raised on grass and natural plant sources, as opposed to the growth hormones, antibiotics and GMO feeds that they are fed today. So, back in the 1700s, prior to the industrial revolution, our ancestors were eating the healthiest kind of food.

Today, more than 10 billion animals are raised each year in factories — ready for slaughter (according to *The Humane Society of the United States*). The animals are enclosed in tight spaces, never see the light of day, and eat fortified GMO feed with regular injections of growth hormones that plump them up at an unnatural rate.

To enhance the flavor and taste of meat, milk and other animal-derived products, animals are pumped with drugs and other hormones that diminish their nutritional value, while incorporating harmful chemicals and drugs that adversely affect the health of those who consume them.[1] For

---

[1] https://www.fda.gov/animal-veterinary/safety-health/antimicrobial-resistance

instance, the introduction of margarine as an alternative for 'heart unhealthy' butter. Harvard Nutrition experts[2] call the idea of trans fats (commonly found in margarine) as the biggest food-processing disaster as it is twice as harmful for your heart as butter and causes about 30,000-100,000 premature heart disease-related deaths on a yearly basis.

In early 2012, the FDA banned the usage of cephalosporin (used in farming) as an antibiotic to raise animal growth. Interesting to note that additives can be used until they are proven to be unsafe! In contrast, the EU requires additives to be proven to be safe before they can be used.

Fruits and Vegetables

Conventionally grown produce can be much lower in antioxidants unlike the antioxidants found in organic fruits and vegetables.[3] Organic fruits and vegetables can deliver between 20 and 40 percent more antioxidants than conventional fruits and vegetables. In addition, the journal

---

[2]https://www.thehealthy.com/nutrition/4-most-harmful-ingredients-in-packaged-foods/
[3] https://well.blogs.nytimes.com/2012/09/04/organic-food-vs-conventional-food

of HortScience which contains a report about the state of American fruits and vegetables shows that the non-organic produce not only tastes worse organic produce but it also contains fewer nutrients[4].

According to Donald R. Davis, a former research associate with the Biochemical Institute at the University of Texas, Austin the average vegetable that is available in the supermarket is somewhere between 5% to 40% lower in minerals which include magnesium, iron, calcium, and zinc. This shows a considerable decline in the nutritional value than that harvested just 50 years ago.

Studies have linked the idea of a long term pesticide usage and consumption to several diseases like respiratory concerns, multiple types of cancers and mental challenges like depression. An increased usage of pesticides, herbicides, chemical fertilizers and other chemicals has disrupted the quality and composition of the soil, making it ill fit for growing plants that deliver a nutritional punch. In order to kill the intended victim – insects etc., we use chemical

---

[4] https://www.motherearthnews.com/natural-health/good-calories-bad-calories-zmaz08onzgoe

pesticides that are heavily composed of toxic ingredients and heavy metals like arsenic, copper, sulfates, lead, and mercury. These directly affect the nervous system. These can cause damage to the vital organs as well. As a result, human beings fall victim to these toxins. However, there is a very little we can do to control agricultural concern especially because we can't control use of the highly used pesticides.

Did you know…Pesticides, to a certain extent, have been used in organic farming[5] as well? What needs to be taken into consideration here are the two different kinds of pesticides, synthetic and natural. There are 900 synthetic pesticides in use for conventional farming in contrast to 25 organic approved synthetic pesticides for organic farming. Organic farming mainly relies on natural pesticides that are not toxic, unlike lab-created, synthetic pesticides.

Processed Foods

It's interesting how packaged and processed foods have drastically changed our lifestyle. The 1950s marked the

---

[5] https://www.ecowatch.com/pesticides-organic-farming-2292594453.html

emerging trend of fast foods, and now, just more than half a century later, nearly 80 percent of processed foods contain genetically modified ingredients. They are packed with artificial flavors, sweeteners, colors, and preservatives; that makes them last longer; at the expense of world health. Just the other day I was looking at a package of tofu. When I looked closer to the package I read that it wasn't really tofu at all. It was a synthetically modified tofu-like product.

Consuming Too Many Processed Foods: The Consequences to your Health

In our society of immediate gratification, we are all looking for a quick fix for a meal – all of us are in this race to achieve the most in the least possible time. The option of readymade meals, packaged dinners, frozen pizzas, and canned & processed foods offer us a quick way to fill our growling bellies with the least amount of effort. However, while we save our precious 'time' not preparing or cooking our food, we are in fact, compromising our health. Is time, so much more precious to you than good health? Do you make time for other activities – catching up with your favorite series, going out to dinner at your favorite restaurant, checking your phone every couple of minutes, going out and having fun – then why not take out an hour or less to prepare your own meals? I am not talking about gourmet cooking, but just the simple act of tossing a salad with fresh greens, making your own lasagna (instead of using the readymade frozen option that has many additives and preservatives that allow it to last longer), and opting for other healthier choices that will promote your good health.

You might choose to look the other way when someone tries to push you in the right direction, but it is important that we realize the fact that proper nutrition is what makes us healthy.

Eating Processed Foods – The consumption of processed foods can lead to major health issues. Highly processed foods are becoming a major trend in the world and the dependency on such foods is inevitable. Cereals, canned fruit, canned vegetable are just a few foods that fill the inner shelves of grocery stores.

Did you know there are food scientists whose primary job it is, is to make food taste better in a way that almost makes it addictive? With the right combination of food additives, you may have a hard time having just one. Whether it is eating a bag of chips, drinking carbonated beverages, sweets and chocolates or other forms of comfort foods. Processed and canned foods tend to have additives, in order to add to their shelf life. There are many additives the food industry uses. A few of the highly used additives are food dyes, high fructose corn syrup, trans fats and sodium nitrate. Artificial food dyes are suspected to cause increased hyperactivity in children. Also, the dye Yellow No. 5 has been thought to worsen asthma symptoms. (In the 1970s, the FDA famously banned Red Dye No. 2 after some studies found that large doses could cause cancer in rats).

High fructose corn syrup is another highly used additive. Studies have made the connection between high fructose corn syrup and the risk of obesity and Type 2 diabetes. Trans fats are believed to increase the risk of heart disease and Type 2 diabetes. Sodium nitrate is found in the preservation of meats and is suspected to cause gastric cancer.

Preservatives – When you visit your local grocery store to buy a jar of peanut butter and jelly, do you really know how long the jars have been sitting on that shelf that you eventually end up buying? A long shelf life indicates the presence of preservatives and there is nothing good about a long shelf life. Of course, there are natural ways of preserving foods, but they don't make it last for years as opposed to the 'long term' expiry date that is present on processed foods labels. Many preservatives, like sulfites, which serve their purpose of stopping the discoloration of edibles, have had connections with allergies and asthma concerns[6] Whether it is sauces, jams, jellies, nut butter, pickles, or anything else sitting on that shelf, it is made with harmful preservatives that will make it survive a couple years, or more on the shelf. Have you ever seen what happens to the same food out in the open without the likes of sulfites? How long do they last? A week or two at best. Well, that's the kind of food you should be eating – without preservatives.

Artificial Colors– Colors have been used in the food industry to make them more appealing and attractive. Kids often choose the bright colored packaged biscuits and chips when they don't know the kind of flavor that they want. But did you know that only seven food colors have been approved by the FDA?[7] But even those are now considered

---

[6] https://www.ecowatch.com/pesticides-organic-farming-2292594453.html
[7]

to increase the symptoms of ADHD and other focus disorders in children. The caramel color – most commonly used in sodas – has been found to be carcinogenic. It's high time for us to realize that we are playing with our lives and jeopardizing our health by eating processed foods. It is important to understand our bodies and keep in mind the nutrition it needs and deserves. A basic argument here would be that the healthier your food source, the healthier you will be.

Food dyes found in processed foods are:

- FD&C Blue No. 2 (indigotine)
- FD&C Green No. 3 (fast green FCF)
- FD&C Red No. 3 (erythrosine)
- FD&C Red No. 40 (allura red AC)
- FD&C Yellow No. 5 (tartrazine)
- FD&C Yellow No. 6 (sunset yellow)
- Orange B (restricted to use in hot dog and sausage casings)

It's important to note that collectively these are associated with allergies, brain tumors, bladder and

---

https://www.fda.gov/ForIndustry/ColorAdditives/ColorAdditiveInventories/ucm115641.html

testicular cancer, thyroid tumors, adrenal tumors, kidney tumors, ADD/ADHD and hypersensitivity reactions.

You Are What You Eat

You might have heard it somewhere, but *you are what you eat*. Whatever goes into our mouths, gets digested and absorbed into the bloodstream. From there it goes into our cells, tissues, and organs, forming an indistinguishable part of our body. It's essential to pay attention to what you eat and the kind of eating habits that you develop or re-develop. Whether you are a junk food enthusiast or someone who thrives on natural produce, there are certain parts of your body that may react adversely with your dietary intake.

These reactions may be due to foods that have pesticide residue, toxic chemicals, food additives, preservatives, or artificial color or flavoring. Even though pesticides are used to kill pests they can be very harmful. The residue of pesticides remains on the food surface and may affect your health when you consume them.

Diseases

A typical grocery store has a higher percentage of their square footage dedicated to processed and canned foods, packaged dinners and frozen items, as compared to fresh vegetables, fruits, and meat. When you're shopping, keep to the perimeter of the store as this is where you'll find the fewest processed foods.

Following are some diseases and illnesses that may be triggered by the foods that we consume:

Cancer

The most common types of cancer include that of the breast, prostate, cervical, colorectal, lungs, liver and stomach. Microwave popcorn, canned goods, grilled red meat, refined sugar, salted, pickled, and smoked foods, soda and carbonated beverages, white flour, farmed fish and hydrogenated oils are among some of the most common cancer-causing foods.[8] In addition to the above-mentioned foods, studies have also found that foods labeled as light, fat-

---

[8]http://www.natuoil.com/wp-content/uploads/2014/02/2.-Proposed-Ban-of-Trans-Fats.pdf

free or diet are also among foods that may be causing cancer. The common element in all these ingredients / foods is the fact that the food structure is altered in one way or another through artificial means. For example, hydrogenated oils undergo a chemical process which turns the oil into trans fats. This process helps manufacturers save money. White flour undergoes extensive processing and refining which removes the most nutritious part of the grain, GMOs have a modified genetic makeup, carbonated beverages contain artificial flavors and colorings, just to name a few.

Hydrogenated oils are commonly used to preserve processed foods and stabilize an extended shelf life. Foods containing hydrogenated oils can increase levels of LDL (bad cholesterol), while decreasing HDL (good cholesterol), and may harm your heart health. Safer oils to add to your pantry are: organic butter, coconut, palm or extra virgin olive oil.

DDT and Brain Disorders

Studies have shown that Alzheimer's and Parkinson's disease have a very high chance of developing when exposed to DDT, which is a chemical found[9] in many pesticides. Although DDT has been banned in the US since 1972, people are still at risk of coming into contact with it in different ways. You can be exposed to DDT by buying foods that have been imported from countries like Northern Africa, South America, and Asia where DDT is still used to this day. *NOTE: DDT takes many years, even decades to break down naturally, so it remains in the soil.*

But DDT is just one example of harmful pesticides, there are other chemicals in pesticides, herbicides and processed foods in general that have harmful effects on the brain's structure and function.

Herbicides such as Paraquat and pesticide such as Rotenone have been widely linked to Parkinson's disease, lung scarring, liver, kidney and heart failure.

ADHD

ADHD or Attention Deficit Hyperactivity Disorder is a behavioral disorder that mainly affects children. The

---

[9] https://time.com/4139/the-pesticide-on-your-fruit-may-lead-to-parkinsons/

symptoms of ADHD can be triggered by the consumption of certain foods – for example: eggs, sugar, gluten, food dyes.[10] Dairy products, such as yogurt, cheese and ice cream, as well as, sugar, chocolate, coffee, frozen pizza, chips, red meat, soda, boxed fruit juices, corn, squash, and fast foods are on the list of foods that should be avoided by ADHD patients. Ingredients that can exacerbate ADHD symptoms can include preservatives, artificial flavors, and coloring, and any processed foods. It's best to stick with whole foods but of course, checking with your physician before making any changes to your or your child's diet is really important.

Food Intolerance and Allergies

Food intolerance and sensitivities are typically more common than food allergies. Food intolerance is caused by food that can't be properly digested. For example, I'm sure you've heard of lactose intolerance. It happens when the body lacks a specific enzyme, lactase, which works to break down lactose in order to allow proper digestion.

---

[10] http://abcnews.go.com/Health/Allergies/adhd-food-allergy-case-restricting-diet/story?id=12832958

Some food sensitivities include gluten, wheat, sensitivity to sulfites, dyes, additives and other preservatives found in processed, frozen or boxed foods. Symptoms of food sensitivities may vary but are all symptoms are related to the digestive system, such as gas, bloating, diarrhea, constipation, nausea, and cramping. The following food additives may cause some of these adverse reactions:

- ❖ MSG (monosodium glutamate) is used as a flavor enhancer and can cause headaches.

- ❖ Nitrates can cause itching and skin rashes. Normally processed meats are high in nitrates and nitrites.

- ❖ Some colorings, particularly red can cause severe problems and inflammation.

Sulfites, used for preserving and enhancing foods are commonly used in wines and have been linked to respiratory problems. Sulfites can have various adverse effects on our bodies such as follows:

- ❖ Digestive disorders

- ❖ Lung irritations

- ❖ Impedes absorption of Vitamin B

❖ Nausea

❖ Asthma

Food allergies, on the other hand, are triggered by a response mediated by the immune system. These allergies can be more severe than insensitivities or intolerance. The most common symptoms of food allergies include hives, eczema, and diarrhea, and vomiting, runny nose, blood in stools, skin rashes, and wheezing. Different foods trigger different allergic reactions in different individuals depending on their immune system.

The U.S. Centers for Disease Control[11] state that there are eight types of food which cause about 90 percent of food allergies; peanuts, wheat, eggs, fish, cow's milk, soy foods, crustacean shellfish (which includes crab, scallops, prawns, shrimp, and lobsters) and tree nuts (which include pecans, hazelnuts, pistachios, almonds, walnuts, Brazil nuts, chestnuts, and cashews). So although we are not literally what we eat, our bodies absorb everything we put into it. When choosing foods, opt for the healthier choices. Chapter

---

[11] https://www.fda.gov/Food/ResourcesForYou/Consumers/ucm079311.html

3 provides some of the cleaner, nutritious foods.

Diet Plan or Lifestyle

The modern health landscape is ruled by a plethora of diet plans that each focus on specific nutritional guidelines. With the advancement in both science and technology, the nutritional world is also shaped and influenced by their development. The food of today is not the same as that of decades ago – what our ancestors consumed and what was, without a doubt, the secret of their health and beauty.

But today, all of us are striving to strike that perfect balance between our diet and lifestyle to remain fit and healthy. Many of you have probably tried one or another form of dieting – whether it's low-carb-high-protein, low-fat or any of the other nutritional approaches that incorporate all or particular food groups based on dietary guidelines. The thing is, we all are struggling to be the healthiest version of ourselves – both on the inside and out. Achieving and maintaining a healthy weight and body is the strongest driving force for people seeking a diet that supports their individual bodies and lifestyle. The following are some of the popular trends supported by science[12] and research that have been adopted by nutritionists and diet enthusiasts for the purpose of losing weight without compromising on health.

Atkins diet

This nutritional approach focuses on controlling insulin – a hormone that regulates glucose – levels in the body by following a low-carb diet. The basic idea is to prevent the insulin spikes that mainly occur as a result of eating refined carbs and sugar. This increases blood glucose. In turn, insulin levels increase, enabling the body to store the excess glucose as fat, making it less likely for it to be used as an energy source later.

So, people who follow the Atkins diet avoid processed and refined carbs and eat more of protein and fat. This decreases your appetite and you remain full for longer. The Atkins diet has been shown to lower the risk of certain diseases and maintaining blood pressure, sugar, insulin and cholesterol levels in the body. It is also proven to be highly

---

[12] https://www.healthline.com/nutrition/9-weight-loss-diets-reviewed

successful in reducing belly fat, the most harmful fat that is responsible for the famous potbelly, beer belly or the spare tire.

Vegetarian diet

A vegetarian diet comprises of only plant-based food sources, and also includes eggs, dairy, and honey. Vegetarians often have lower body weight, are less susceptible to diseases and have a longer life expectancy than meat-eaters.[13] However, those who are new to being vegetarians need to watch out for the balance of a healthy diet.

There are many benefits which are associated with being a vegetarian but it is not simply to cut the meat, poultry, and seafood from the daily menu. Animal products do offer nutrients that support growth, body functions, and a healthy immune system. These nutrients are necessary to be consumed from other sources after you quit eating meat so that you can cater to all your body's nutritional needs. For example, you can fulfill your protein intake from a lot of

---

[13] https://www.sparkpeople.com/resource/nutrition_articles.asp?id=1530

plant-based sources. Vegetarians should be careful that they have sources that provide vital nutrients like protein, Vitamin B12, Iron, Zinc and Omega 3. [14]

Vegan diet

In 1944, Donald Watson created the vegan diet which eliminates all animal-based food sources, including dairy, eggs, honey and all animal-derived products such as gelatin, whey, and albumin. A study done in 2013 by the Loma Linda University indicated that vegans are shown to have lower body weight and BMI as compared to those that follow other diets. They have a lower risk of developing type 2 diabetes and heart disease.

However, a vegan diet is not very effective for weight loss as compared to other diets when matched for calories. In many cases, vegans are deficient in various nutrients – vitamin D and B12, iron, calcium, zinc, and omega-3 fatty acids – due to the elimination of all animal food sources. But these nutritional deficiencies may be overcome by

---

[14] https://www.health.harvard.edu/staying-healthy/becoming-a-vegetarian

incorporating foods high in these nutrients into their diets.

Raw food diet

A raw food diet contains plant-based food and drinks that are organic and unprocessed. Seventy-five percent of the daily caloric intake of this diet comprises of uncooked food. Many raw foodists are also vegans, choosing to eliminate all animal food sources from their diet.

Mediterranean diet

South-European in origin, this diet approach focuses on plants as the main sources of dietary fats, such as nuts, olive oil, whole grains, and seeds. It also includes moderate to small amounts of dairy; such as cheese and yogurt, poultry, red meat, and wine. About one-third of the Mediterranean diet comprises of fat, however, the saturated fats are less than 8 percent of the caloric intake. The diet is proven to be beneficial in lowering the risk of heart disease, stroke and may also reduce the risk of Parkinson's or Alzheimer's disease.

Paleo Diet

The paleo diet follows the diet of our hunter-gatherer ancestors, as it is believed that most modern diseases occur due to the consumption of grains, dairy, and processed foods. When following a paleo diet, people are encouraged to eat more of whole foods, vegetables, fruits, lean meat, as well as nuts and seeds, while eliminating dairy, sugar, grains and processed foods. This diet seems to be effective at reducing the risk of heart disease by lowering cholesterol, blood sugar, and blood pressure.

The idea behind healthy eating is to find a regime, stick to it, and ensure that it is the best fit according to your individual needs. Depending on your food sensitivity or allergy, you can choose a diet or lifestyle that best suits your palate.

The common ground between all these diet approaches is the fact that all are developed on a one size fits all approach. It's important to strive to cut down the unhealthy components of today's foods – GMOs, factory-farmed animals, and processed and non-organic foods – while incorporating the components of healthy food, such as wholesome fresh produce, grass-fed meat, and organically grown produce. Sticking to a natural way of living and eating foods that are as unique as you are. It is about time that we realize the fact that we are endangering ours, as well as our children's lives by choosing the easier and faster way of consuming food. Remember, *nothing good has ever come easy* and the same goes for eating well and remaining healthy.

In a nutshell, one has to be on the lookout of all the foods that he/she consumes because your gut is responsible for all your health. It controls and influences all the functions of your body and hence has a strong influence on the operations of your body. Your gut health, if gone bad, can impose a major threat to your health. This is going to form the basis of the next chapter in which we will take a detailed look at the gut health.

Keep in mind that whatever diet you choose has to be healthy enough for your gut to accept. Gut health is essential in promoting a healthy lifestyle. A combination of fiber along with healthy pro-biotics keeps the gut healthy. But, much like most diets, promotion of a healthy gut is also not a one size fits all program. One source of fiber may be beneficial for person X but might not work on person Z. In the next chapter, on gut health, we will discuss the intricacies of gut health and how it is essential in overall healthy living.

Chapter 2
Gut Health

"Gut health is the key to overall health."

-Kris Carr

The World Health Organization defines *'health'* as the absence of any sort of illness or disease in a particular part of the human or animal body. In this regard, if one were to define gut health it would mean the absence of any illnesses or diseases related to our gut. The term 'Gut health' has been used extensively in medical literature over time and by various food industrialists. Gut health demands focus on the gastrointestinal (GI) tract which include effective digestion and absorption of food.

This concept still remains ambiguous from a scientific point of view. It cannot be precisely defined and measured. Any GI barrier impairment can develop the risk of developing infectious, inflammatory, and functional GI diseases. It could also trigger extra-intestinal diseases that are related to immune-mediated and metabolic disorders. The methods used to assess, improve and maintain gut health-related GI functions remain of significant interest in preventive medicine.[15]

Effects of Poor Gut Health
Inefficient Absorption

It's essential to maintain a proper and balanced diet in order to have balanced bacteria in your body and once your gut health is unstable, absorption becomes difficult.[16]

The gastrointestinal tract which comprises of mouth, stomach, small and large intestines contribute towards the nutrients that your body absorbs. Approximately 92 to 97% of the consumed nutrients include:

- ❖ Minerals
- ❖ Carbohydrates
- ❖ Vitamins
- ❖ Fats
- ❖ Fibers
- ❖ Proteins

---

[15] https://bmcmedicine.biomedcentral.com/articles/10.1186/1741-7015-9-24
[16] https://www.livestrong.com/article/436603-in-which-digestive-organ-are-nutrients-absorbed/

All these nutrients are absorbed through the GI tract. The digestion process begins in your mouth and extends down through your colon. Enzymes are found in human saliva, which helps with breaking down the food into particles and eventually speeds up the digestion process. Each specific organ has a distinctive approach dissolving the food through enzymes and ultimately are absorbed by the intestinal walls.

Without this absorption, the body could be deprived of essential nutrients like calcium, magnesium, iron, chloride, sodium, and zinc. The lack of proper nutrients in the body can result in malabsorption syndrome.

'Malabsorption syndrome' is due to inadequate nutrients being absorbed from your food into the bloodstream. With malabsorption, the small intestine is unable to absorb certain nutrients which can include a list of macronutrients to micronutrients such as proteins, carbohydrates, fats, vitamins, and minerals. The possible causes of malabsorption syndrome include:

❖ Damaged intestine, i.e. from any severe infection, inflammation or surgery.

❖ Prolonged usage of antibiotics.

❖ Other medical conditions contributing to human health such as celiac disease, Crohn's disease, chronic pancreatitis, or cystic fibrosis.

❖ Lactose intolerance or deficiency of lactose in blood.

❖ Certain congenital issues that are there from birth, such as biliary atresia (when the bile ducts don't develop normally and prevent the flow of bile from the liver).

❖ Diseases of the gallbladder, liver, or pancreas.

❖ Parasitic diseases.

❖ Radiation therapies that include being exposed to radioactive particles or laser beams may injure the lining of the intestine.

❖ Certain drugs that may injure the lining of the intestine, such as tetracycline, colchicine, or cholestyramine.

This condition is also exacerbated if your stomach is not able to produce adequate enzymes in order to digest foods.

Impacts of Gut Health on Your Immune System

Our gut wall houses 70 percent of the cells that contribute towards making our immune system work. Diseases such as allergies, arthritis, autoimmune diseases (irritable bowel syndrome, acne, and chronic fatigue), mood disorders, autism, dementia, and cancer are usually not attributed to digestive problems but your gut is actually responsible for it. In order to repair your health, you should begin with your gut because it is a trigger point for all your health problems.[17]

The importance of your gut includes: breaking down your food, absorbing nutrients and eliminating toxins. Considering the kind of functions that your gut has to perform it's clear that it has to function seamlessly in order to guarantee an excellent immune system. Healthy gut flora is crucial for optimal gut health. Your gut serves as a habitat for over 500 bacteria species weighing up to three pounds. Too many bad florae may have a negative impact on your

---

[17] https://www.ecowatch.com/how-good-gut-health-can-boost-your-immune-system-1882013643.html

health. Your gut nervous system (known as the enteric nervous system) contributes to your health by acting as your second brain. Research shows that the gut-brain connection plays a massive role in determining not only the gastrointestinal function but also the state of feeling and intuitive decision making.

Other than the brain, your gut is the only organ that has its own nervous system. Your gut contains about 30 neurotransmitters—your brain contains between 30 to 40 neurotransmitters. If we just talk about your small intestine, it consists of as many neurons as your spinal cord. Your gut nerve cells can produce 95 percent of the serotonin in your body, it's important to ensure your gut is functioning at optimum capacity.

Gut imbalances open doors for many new diseases and disorders such as functional and gastrointestinal disorders, anxiety and depression. Focus on ingesting whole foods, eat more fiber and eat / drink fermented foods.

In addition to this, your gut has to get rid of all the toxins that are produced as a by-product of your metabolism. This is usually dumped by your liver through bile. Limiting alcohol, drinking more water, reducing sugar intake and eating antioxidant rich foods will help with the elimination of toxins.

Disrupts Your Digestive Health

Having a healthy gut means that you have control over your entire health because an unhealthy gut is not only restricted to problems like being annoyed or bloating or heartburn but it practically controls your whole body.[18] Your gut connects to everything that happens in your body. People with chronic health issues may resolve their issues by fixing their gut.

In order to help heal your gut there are several steps you can take:

- ❖ Eat whole, unprocessed foods: kefir, miso, apple cider vinegar, berries, bananas, oatmeal.
- ❖ Eliminate foods you're sensitive to.
- ❖ Treat any infections or overgrowth of yeast.
- ❖ Replenish your digestive enzymes: papaya, pineapple, mango, honey and bananas.

---

[18] https://3rdopinion.us/functional-medicine/gut-digestive-health/

❖ Rebuild your rain forest of friendly bacteria with probiotics: kefir, yogurt, milk and cheese with added probiotics, kimchi, kombucha.

❖ Consume good fat: avocado, hard cheese, fatty fish.

❖ Heal your gut lining with foods high in glutamin: celery, kale, fermented foods, spinach, carrots. etc.

❖ Eat foods high in Zinc: meat, shellfish, legumes.

Your gut determines what nutrients will be absorbed and what toxins will be flushed out. Simply put, gut health can be defined by optimal digestion, absorption, and assimilation of food.

Many diseases that seem totally unrelated to the gut, such as eczema or psoriasis or arthritis, are actually caused by gut problems. By focusing on your gut you can get better.[19]

Keeps You from Your Desired Weight

An uncontrollable condition of weight increase can actually point towards the fact that you need to take care of your digestive system i.e. your gut health.[20] Poor digestion

---

[19] https://3rdopinion.us/functional-medicine/gut-digestive-health/
[20] https://www.livestrong.com/article/496197-poor-digestion-weight-gain/

can lead to weight gain which is actually a consequence of your digestive system's inability to properly break down foods. This once again leads to a condition where your body is unable to absorb adequate nutrients and eliminate the waste and toxins in your body which in turn causes constipation and bloating. The disruption of the pattern of proper absorption and dissolving of food particles in the form of nutrients becomes a hurdle for a healthy metabolism. And when your metabolism does not function properly, it slows down the process of digestion of food which turns into saturated unhealthy fats, staying in the body, causing fatigue or obesity.

According to a claim by Mayo Clinic:

"Researchers have identified a difference in the types of bacteria found in a lean person's gut versus those that live in the gut of some who is obese. The amount of energy is small, but researchers wonder if over time this could be a factor in weight maintenance."[21]

---

[21] http://www.chicagotribune.com/lifestyles/health/sns-201805101135--tms--mayoclnctnmc-b20180510-20180510-story.html

Weakens Your Brain

The mind affects our gut and vice versa. There have been a number of studies conducted throughout the world that have proven the relationship the gut and brain. In 2011, British Scientists tested both rats and human subjects by giving them both probiotics. They called in the [human] subjects a month later and saw a massive decrease in the levels of anxiety, distress, anger, and depression. More recently, research from Oxford concluded that supplements specifically designed to cater to GI bacteria work on improving anxiety levels. After the subjects were provided with the supplements, they tended to pay less attention to negativity over time.

Gut health over the years has been overlooked, but in recent times the gut is gaining attention. There are certain ways that gut health can be improved. Of course, every person is different and needs to be treated differently but there are basics that can help most people with mild gut concerns.

"Scientists are now revealing that there is a strong link between what happens in the gut and the brain. The bacteria

that reside in the gut appear to play an important role and are able to communicate with the central nervous system notably through neural, endocrine and immune pathways. By influencing the balance and types of bacteria present, studies show that it may be possible to lower stress, affect cognition/brain processes and mood. "[22]

- Dr. Helene M. Savignac Ph.D., Brain Research Manager

What Strengthens Your Gut?

Nature has been kind enough to give us foods that can not only eliminate any unwanted diseases from our gut but also make it much stronger. These foods, for the most part, are foods that contain probiotics which is basically good bacteria that assist in developing a healthy gut. However, some of these foods also contain prebiotics which a healthy gut feeds on:

---

[22] https://www.sociedelic.com/why-and-how-your-state-of-mind-affects-your-gut-and-vice-versa/

Apple Cider Vinegar	Miso
Kombucha	Chocolate
Mango	Kimchi
Yogurt	Wild Salmon
Coconut Oil	4R Treatment

Apple Cider Vinegar

Whenever anyone is looking for a resolution related to the stomach, Apple Cider Vinegar always makes it to the list. It can be called a magic food because it promotes the creation of hydrochloric acid inside of our bodies, which in turn helps in the digestion of all the macro-nutrients effectively.

It relieves symptoms of irritable bowel syndrome and acid reflux owing to all the probiotics and amino acids that it contains. Apple Cider Vinegar can also aid weight loss. While focusing on the usage of Apple Cider Vinegar for the improvement of one's gut health, the intake of glass (8 Oz) of water mixed with a 1-3 teaspoons of apple cider vinegar before a meal can improve digestion.[23] It can improve

---

[23] https://bodyunburdened.com/use-apple-cider-vinegar-improve-digestion/

nutrient assimilation by increasing HCl production. You can start with 1 teaspoon and you can see what impacts it has on your health.

Kombucha

Kombucha tastes slightly acidic, with a fresh, sparkling taste. However, there is no denying the fact that it's packed with probiotics, making it ideal for gut health. Kombucha is made out of fermented tea, bacteria, sugar, and yeast and is a perfect choice to have in order to have a healthy gut. The greatest reason why kombucha supports digestion is that it possesses high levels of beneficial acid, probiotics, amino acids, and enzymes.[24] Although Kombucha contains bacteria, that bacteria is healthy. Don't get confused by the term 'healthy bacteria', it means the bacteria which is harmless to human metabolism. In fact, the bacteria that Kombucha contains helps fight the pathogen bacteria in the gut.

---

[24] https://draxe.com/7-reasons-drink-kombucha-everyday/

Mango

Mangoes can play a positive role in shaping your digestive system for the good. It helps in keeping the good bacteria alive in your body. Recently, the Oklahoma State University concluded in a study that one mango a day could keep an unhealthy gut away. Mangoes contain bioactive compounds, and if consumed in moderation can control blood sugar and help reduce body fat, which again is a good sign for improving your gut.

Mangoes can fight inflammation in your gut due to the presence of beneficial compounds like vitamins, minerals, and phenolic acids. Mangoes are helpful in treating chronic constipation. An increase in consuming mangoes guarantees less severe symptoms of inflammation in the gut. Along with this, mangoes help your gut to absorb a great deal of iron. Iron deficiency is considered one of the most widespread nutritional deficiency in the world.

With the help of iron, the body directs the red blood cells to carry oxygen and circulate around the body. This, in turn, boosts the immune system and its cognitive performance. Researchers found that those who regularly ate mangoes consumed higher amounts of dietary fiber, vitamins B6 and

C, magnesium, and potassium. They also ate less added sugar and sodium. Mangoes can help a great deal to bolster our body's natural defense and improve our gut health which will have a lasting effect on the overall health of our body.[25]

Yogurt

This is a rather well-known food when it comes to gut health and digestive problems. Both dairy and soy yogurt contains a high number of probiotics. These probiotics are vital when it comes to removing toxins, fungus, and bad bacteria. This, in turn, may help relieve symptoms of irritable bowel syndrome.

Coconut Oil

Recently, the benefits of coconut oil keep emerging. Coconut Oil has proven to be an important food as far as digestion is concerned. It has caprylic as well as lauric acids that help to kill all bad bacteria and also helps in maintaining a stable level of acidity in your stomach.

---

[25] https://www.mindbodygreen.com/0-26402/a-guthealthy-fruit-that-fights-inflammation-that-you-can-eat-all-year-round.html

Miso

A good tasting soup-like meal Miso is something that is incredibly rich in probiotics, which makes it a very good choice for the treatment of intestinal disorders. Apart from this, Miso also serves as a good source of fiber and proteins. Both of them are gut-friendly, and help our bodies to stay healthy. However, the consumption should be limited because of the high sodium content in Miso.

Chocolate

This might be the best way to keep your gut clean and clear. Organic chocolate and cocoa are a great source of prebiotic as well as probiotics. Chocolate can contain protein, vitamin E, calcium, phosphorus, magnesium, iron, copper, and antioxidants. Even though most available chocolates have preservatives and extra sugar, the natural and organic kind and especially dark chocolate with high cocoa content can be an excellent treat for your gut.

Cocoa, which is the main ingredient of chocolate, possesses the beneficial characteristics which enable our body to absorb the nutrients from the chocolate. We need our tiny microbial passengers to break complex molecules into smaller components. This would not be possible for our bodies to perform otherwise. Our body can make use of the health-promoting molecules in cocoa. In addition to this, the gut bacteria also enjoy this food. It produces an even greener effect on our health.

Kimchi

Kimchi is a low-calorie, high fiber, and nutrient-packed side dish. It is a storehouse of a range of vitamins such as vitamin A, vitamin B1, vitamin B2, and vitamin C. It is also rich in essential amino acids and minerals such as iron, calcium, and selenium. It's beneficial for cases like bowel pain, irritation, leaky guts, and inflammation. Not only does it have soothing effects, but also happens to be incredibly rich when it comes to probiotics and does a decent job of keeping food and other particles moving inside of your digestive tract.

Wild Salmon

Here the emphasis lies on the word WILD. A salmon caught wild has almost three times the amount of nutrients than the one usually found at supermarkets and contains protein, selenium, niacin, vitamin B12, vitamin B6, and riboflavin. This wild salmon naturally possesses an insane amount of omega-3 fatty acids which help curb the inflammation and heal the gut in its worst states. It also prevents any other episodes of inflammation that may take place in the future.

4R Treatment

There are quite a few natural resources and foods that contribute to building a healthy and stable digestive system. As mentioned earlier, it is important to take notice of the fact that these are general guidelines and do not cater to individual gut concerns. Gut health requires a lot of consideration in order to maintain a healthy lifestyle since it forms the focal point of the health of a person's body. In regards to this, many practitioners opt for a particular program that is called the *4R treatment plan/program.* The program may have different names but it focuses on optimizing health, specifically health concerns regarding the gut. This program focuses on four Rs.

* Removing excess

* Replacing deficiency

❖ Repopulation of the gut

❖ Repairing the integrity of the gut

Removing Excess

The first step of the 4R treatment is removing excess which involves removing any particle or excessive stressors that harm the GI tract. First and foremost, the stressor that seems to disturb the GI tract is alcohol. Alcohol has been proven time and again to cause problems like heartburn and acid reflux.

It forces contact with the gut lining for absorption in the bloodstream which can lead to a gut disturbance or diarrhea. Alcohol has also been proven to contribute to a leaky gut, which basically refers to the inability of the gut lining to prevent toxins from getting into your bloodstream.

Organizations like the NHS have recommended a reduction of alcohol for people experiencing acid reflux symptoms to determine whether the symptoms improve. Making small changes, in this regard could be the way to go. A healthy gut is important when you're trying to maintain a healthy body. The second thing that needs to be addressed, is reducing your intake of refined carbohydrates. Refined carbohydrates sources are bread, pizza crust, muffins, breakfast cereals to name a few. Think of it as eliminating processed foods. For breakfast try a breakfast quinoa, crustless quiche or overnight breakfast in bed. *(See recipe section for more).*

Eggs, salmon, clams and chicken are all high in vitamin B12. Some studies show that vitamin B12 deficiency may cause tiredness, loss of appetite, constipation or weakness so increasing your diet with foods high in B12 may also result in having a little more energy.

Thirdly, we need to work towards eliminating stress. Here, when we say stress we are referring to the Sympathetic Nervous System that's activated every time the body is set for a challenge or for a 'fight-flight' response. Surprisingly, stress can cause spasms in your esophagus which can increase stomach acid and indigestion. Carrots, eggs, avocados, and bananas are all good sources that will help your body to eliminate stress.

Replacing Deficiency

To make sure that your deficiencies are dealt with there are certain nutrients that the body needs to replace. The replacement of these nutrients needs to be maintained for proper digestion of food. Following is a short list of vegetables and fruit and their primary health benefits.

Vegetables

100 g	Vitamins	Minerals	Main Health Benefits
Brussel Sprouts	A, Thiamine, Riboflavin, Niacin, B6, C, E, K, Pantothenic Acid, Folate	Calcium, Iron, Potassium	Eye health, Nervous system, Red blood cells, Cancer and Diabetes prevention
Kale	A, C, K, Folate	Calcium, Potassium	Eye health, Immune health, Good blood clotting, Cell health, Bone health, Cancer prevention
Broccoli	B Complex, Riboflavin, Pantothenic Acid, B6, Folate, A, C, K	Iron, Zinc, Phosphorous, Calcium, Potassium	Energy, Growth and development, Protein and carb breakdown, Prevents UV (sun) Skin damage, Prevents osteoarthritis, Cell and DNA

			protection, Cancer prevention, Detoxification, Heart health
Cauliflower	C, K, B6, Thiamine, Niacin, Folate, Biotin	Potassium, Manganese	Immune system, Collagen production, Good blood clotting, Blood pressure regulation, Bone health, Metabolism
Asparagus	A, B6, C, Folate, Thiamine, Riboflavin, Niacin, K	Calcium, Zinc, Magnesium, Potassium	Eye health, Immune booster, Prevents kidney stones, Diabetes prevention
Spinach	A, C, K, B6, Folate	Calcium, Iron, Magnesium, Potassium	Eye health, Brain function, Bone health, Cancer prevention, Asthma prevention, Lowers blood pressure
Celery	C, K, Pantothenic Acid	Potassium, Manganese, Sodium	Healthy skin, teeth, ligaments, Immune function, Heart function, Cancer prevention, Joint pain
Cucumber	A, K	Calcium, Potassium, Phosphorus, Molybdenum	Eye health, Bone health, Metabolism, Immune function

White Onion	C, B6, Folic Acid	Potassium, Iron, Phosphorus, Calcium	Collagen production, Immune function, Tissue growth and repair, Cell health
Carrots	A, C, K	Magnesium, Phosphorus, Potassium	Eye health, Collagen production, Lower lung cancer risk, Good blood clotting

Fruit

100 g	Vitamins	Minerals	Main Health Benefits
Blackberries	A, C, E, K, Folate	Copper, Magnesium, Manganese, Potassium	Eye health, Iron absorption, Electrolyte balance, Heart health
Cranberries	A, C, E, K, B, Folate	Calcium, Chromium, Manganese, Copper, Iron, Magnesium, Potassium, Sulphur	Anti-bacterial, Immune function, Heart health, Protein metabolism, Cholesterol control
Pomegranate	B6, C, E, K, Folate, Panthenic Acid	Calcium, Copper, Manganese, Potassium, Phosphorus	Tissue health, Heart health, Iron absorption, Electrolyte balance
Avocado	B6, C, E, K, Folate, Panthenic Acid,	Potassium	Cell repair, Tissue and heart health

	Niacin, Riboflavin		
Pear	C, K Folate	Potassium	Antioxidant, Tissue health, Good clotting, Cell repair and production
Banana	C, B6, B Complex	Potassium	Cell repair, Tissue and heart health, Electrolyte balance
Lemon	A, B Complex, C	Calcium, Copper, Potassium	Eye health, Cell repair, Iron absorption, Detoxification
Apple	A, C, Folate, B Complex	Calcium, Iron, Phosphorus, Potassium, Chromium	Eye health, Tissue health, Blood sugar balance, Anemia prevention, Bone health
Blueberries	C, E, K	Copper, Magnesium, Manganese, Potassium	Iron absorption, Electrolyte balance, Heart health, Detoxification
Oranges	A, C, B Complex	Calcium, Potassium, Phosphorus, Magnesium, Manganese, Selenium, Copper	Eye and tissue health, Immune strength, Bone health, Cancer prevention, Electrolyte balance

In order to find out what you're deficient in, check with your local health care practicioner.

Repopulation of the Gut

Once the replacement has been done, one needs to begin and repopulate the gut with some good bacteria. This is essential in order to have a healthy balance of microflora. These are organisms that reside in the gut and work towards digestion and maintaining a healthy gut. This repopulation can be done by eating several different kinds of food which include foods with pre as well as probiotics.

Pre-biotics: Most of these are plant components that work towards maintaining and enhancing the microflora. These include oligosaccharides along with fructoligosaccharides which are a certain type of carbohydrate that can be found in certain fruits and vegetables. Primary sources include garlic, onions, bananas, and leeks. Another form of prebiotics can be foods with soluble fiber. As the name suggests, it is the fiber that is easily dissolved in water and sources include oatmeal, pears, psyllium, apples, and flaxseed. Finally, prebiotics also have a specific kind of soluble fiber called the Arabinogalactans. Arabinogalactans can protect against infections and help to stimulate the immune system. Sources where you can find this fiber rich complex carbohydrate are, pears, tomatoes, and carrots.

Fermented Foods: These foods were mentioned earlier and include apple cider vinegar, mango, kombucha, kefir, kombucha, miso, and yogurt.

Probiotics: This refers to living bacteria that helps the human body through the process of digestion. Not only do they keep the gut strong, but they also keep it flourishing. These are conveniently available in the form of supplements, however foods like dark chocolate and miso soup, too have proven to be strong probiotics.

Repairing the Integrity of the Gut

It is very important to keep in mind that the gut needs to be repaired just like any other part of your body.

There are a number of things that can be done in order to begin the process of repairing it. Eating whole unprocessed foods is a great start. Food sources include asparagus, avocados, salmon, mushrooms and broccoli. Vitamin D is also important in repairing the gut and can be found in tuna, salmon, mackerel, cheese, egg yolks as well as the sunlight.

Nutrients that can aid a reparation include Omega 3 Fatty Acids, Zinc, Magnesium, and Glutamine. These substances will work towards clearing the gut of bad particles and cleaning up the damage that has been done. Celery, broccoli, asparagus, carrots, blackberries, cranberries and oranges will help you get these nutrients.

Chapter 3
Organic vs. Non-Organic

Organic food has become a popular choice for many people today. However, there is still confusion about its potential benefits. Is organic food better for physical and mental health? Is buying organic food an affordable option for me? This chapter is a guide for these people who want to learn about organic food and its benefits.

What Does 'Organic' Mean?

We've all heard the term 'organic' but what does it really mean? It refers to agricultural products that are grown and processed in a 'more natural' way. The Department for Environment Food and Rural Affairs (DEFRA) states:

'Organic' food is the product of a farming system which avoids the use of man-made fertilizers, pesticides, growth regulators, and livestock feed additives. Irradiation and the use of genetically modified organisms (GMOs) or products produced from or by GMOs are generally prohibited by organic legislation. Organic agriculture is a systems approach to production that is working toward environmentally, socially, and economically sustainable production. Instead, the agricultural systems rely on crop rotation, animal and plant manures, some hand weeding, organic pesticides and biological pest control.'[26]

Understanding GMOs (Genetically Modified Organisms)

There has been an ongoing debate on whether GMOs are safe for health or not. GMOs are engineered in a way that makes them more resistant to herbicides and helps them produce their own insecticides.

GMOs are found in the U.S. crops such as canola, papaya, and squash are present in much of the processed foods that we consume. If the products you consume have soy lecithin or corn syrup in ingredients, chances are that they contain GMOs.

Are GMOs Safe?

The US National Academies of Sciences, Engineering,

------

[26] https://www.bbcgoodfood.com/howto/guide/organic

and Medicine recently released a report that concluded that genetic engineering has no risk as compared to older methods of genetic alteration. However, the Irish Cabinet came up with a proposal "to enable Ireland to prohibit or restrict the cultivation of GMOs in Ireland".

Although the companies that engineer GMOs and the U.S. Food and Drug Administration (FDA) claim that GMOs are safe to use, many food safety advocates disagree. There are no long-term studies conducted on the effects of GMOs on health. While there have been some studies conducted on animals that have proven that GMOs may cause thickening of the digestive tract, slowed brain growth, and internal organ damage, GMOs have also been linked to gastrointestinal problems in humans.

How is Organic Food Different from Non-organic Food?

The basic difference that sets organic food apart from the non-organic one is the way these foods are grown. Organic food is sourced from processes that use no or minimal synthetics such as pesticides and chemical fertilizers. In contrast, non-organic food is produced using synthetics that usually are unhealthy for human consumption. According to research conducted by King's College London, organic food has been found to be more antioxidant-rich. Therefore, it is healthier than the regular (non-organic) food we consume. Moreover, the level of pesticides and toxic metals in organic food sources is far less than those contained by non-organic food. Organic food is richer in both nutrients and taste as compared to its counterpart.

Benefits of Organic Food

The way the food is grown can have major implications for the environment and also has a role to play in a person's emotional and mental health. Organic food is good for everyone. They contains 20-40% more antioxidants as compared to its conventionally-grown counterpart.

Organic food is often fresher as compared to non-organic foods because it does not contain preservatives to make it last longer. Organic produce expire quicker as compared to non-organic foods due to not having waxes or preservatives slathered on them. Eating organic does not always mean that you are eating healthy. It's important to read the labels of organic products before jumping to the conclusion that the product is a healthier option.

Organic Labeling

It is a requirement that composite foods must contain 95% of the ingredients that are organically produced in order to be labeled as organic. EU rules require that regular inspections should be carried out to ensure that the food meets all regulations. The USDA Organic Certification requires that farmers document their processes and have an inspection performed every year. Organic on-site inspections mean inspection of everything from seed sources, soil conditions, crop health, weed and pest management, water systems, etc. Approval from an organic certification body on a regular basis is required and is only given when the production method and labeling requirements are met.

Categories of Organic Product Labels

The label 'organic' is strictly controlled by the United States Department of Agriculture (USDA) and is monitored by the National Organic Program (NOP). It is a certification and can only be used by those who have been inspected and meet federal standards. A farmer can only use this label on their products if there has been a thorough process of inspection at each level of production. Those involved need to have a detailed record and may have to undergo audits at each level of the production chain. There are basically four major categories of this label based on product composition and the labeling specifications, as summarized by the USDA, and are given below.

100% Organic

This label means that the product was primarily made out of all organic ingredients, excluding water and salt. These products cannot use any ingredients listed in the National List of Allowed and Prohibited Substances. These are allowed to use the USDA seal on their panel. Most items in this category are single-ingredient products such as flour or rolled oats.

Organic

This label is used when 95% of the ingredients used were organic, and the product was made using an organic method. The remaining 5% of the products must be non-GMO and must be listed under the National List of non-organic ingredients. The products on this list are certified to best fit into organic agriculture and processing. The authorization of the label also allows the products to carry the USDA seal on their front panel. Most organic products found in grocery stores fall under this category.

Made with Organic Ingredients

These products usually contain somewhere 70 to 90 percent of organic ingredients. The front panel usually lists up to three ingredients. Although these products are certified organic, the USDA seal cannot be used on their packaging. All products must be non-GMO and should have been produced without using sewage sludge or irradiation.

Using this label can be a great stepping stone for companies wanting to go 100% organic or organic. This label is there to show the customer that the company is making an effort. Furthermore, companies can demonstrate their process of going organic onto their websites and let the customers know why they are taking this step.

Specific Ingredient Listings

This category contains products that use less than 70 percent of organic ingredients. These products are allowed to use the word 'organic' in the ingredients panel. However, they are not allowed to use the USDA seal on their packaging. They cannot make a claim about organic certification on their packaging either. Similar to the label 'Made with Organic Ingredients', this label is another way to incorporate the term organic on the label without using all organic ingredients.

Organic Certification

USDA certification is not an easy or cheap task. The facilities at organic-growers must meet the standards. For that, they may have to modify their facilities just to be ready for inspection. There is a strict record-keeping that needs to be in place and the facility can be inspected at any time. Moreover, the organic farmers may have to pay the inspection/certification fee of $400 to $2,000 depending on the size of the facility.

Does Organic Mean Pesticide-Free?

Contrary to popular belief, organic farms do use pesticides as mentioned in chapter one. However, they use naturally-derived pesticides as compared to conventional farms that use synthetic pesticides.

Possible Risks of Pesticides

Our bodies have accumulated pesticides in our system due to exposure to it over the years. This condition is medically known as 'body burden' and could lead to several serious health conditions such as strain on the immune system, rashes, headaches, etc. Some studies show that when a pesticide is consumed unintentionally, it can increase the risk of cancer, even at low doses. These include prostate cancer, breast cancer, brain tumor, lymphoma, and leukemia.

Those most affected by pesticides in our food are children and fetuses because their brain, body, and immune systems are still developing. Exposure to pesticides at an early age can lead to motor dysfunction, immune system harm, autism, behavioral disorder, and developmental delays. Pregnant women may also be affected by pesticides. Pregnant women are more prone to be affected by pesticides and should try to avoid foods with pesticides while pregnant.

Washing and Peeling

Rinsing the products helps to reduce pesticides. Soaking the fruits and vegetables in a vinegar and water mixture for 20 minutes helps in removing pesticides. Peeling can further reduce the pesticides as this removes the top layer of the fruit or vegetable. However, this does not eliminate the pesticides. This may not guarantee total removal of the pesticides but this definitely gives an inner feeling that you are eating clean fruits.

Priority Shopping

Organic food is sometimes more expensive than conventionally grown food. However, you can prioritize where to buy organic food, while balancing the budget. Not all items produced in conventional commercial farms are full of pesticides. The foods high in pesticides should be avoided, choose organic items from the 'Clean 15' list would be a smart choice to make. A non-profit organization named The Environmental Working Group analyzes pesticide testing in the U.S., gives recommendations on the products to purchase, and is updated annually. According to the organization, the following fruits and vegetables, also called the *dirty dozen*, are high in pesticides and it is best to purchase these products from organic sources.

Dirty Dozen (2019)

Peaches	Celery
Apples	Strawberries
Nectarines	Pears
Spinach	Kale
Potatoes	Cherries
Tomatoes	Grapes

The following fruits and vegetables are known as 'Clean 15' since they are generally lower in pesticides, even when produced on a conventional farm.

Clean 15 (2019)

Broccoli	Pineapples
Onions	Corn
Cauliflower	Frozen Sweet Peas

Asparagus	Papayas
Mushrooms	Honeydew Melons
Cabbage	Avocados
Kiwi	Cantaloupes
Eggplant	

Organic Meat

American Health Association have stated that eating organic meat does not carry the same health risks as regular meat and fat. Although most will never have any symptoms from eating non organic meats there are some risks. Risks associated with consuming commercially raised animals range from brain damage, respiratory problems, depression, miscarriage and birth defects.

Organic meat refers to the animals that are raised without any hormones or antibiotics. There are fewer risks associated with organically raised meats. Organic meat may have a higher risk of parasites -- toxoplasmosis. Your risk is reduced when your food is cooked properly and by not consuming any under cooked foods.

Organic Food Buying Tips

❖ Buy fruits that are in season so that you have the freshest food possible. Find out when the products are delivered to your local market. Find a guide to let you know which fruits and vegetables are in season.

❖ Compare the prices offered by the grocery store, the farmer's market, and other venues so that you know the best option available to you to buy organic food at lower prices. Flipp.com or Flipp.ca are great options for finding the best prices at your local markets.

Organic Pesticide Use

Surprisingly organic growers do use pesticides, but they are different pesticides than those used in non-organic farming. There is typically mor labor required in organic farming which is reflected in the price.

Higher Cost of Fertilizer for Organic Crops

Conventional farmers use chemical fertilizers like roundup and sewage sludge because these items are cheap and easy to transport. Organic farmers, on the other hand, use products like Entrust™ which is derived from living organisms. These more natural pesticides may be more expensive and we'll see this reflected in the price at the checkout.

Chapter 4
Food Hacks

Trying to adopt a healthier lifestyle is not an easy thing to do. Even when you know the harm that certain foods and eating habits can cause, changing your regimen often takes more willpower than many of us have. Your body needs time to adjust to a new lifestyle – a sudden change, even if it is for the better, may leave you feeling sick and drained.

During such a time, it can be difficult to figure out how to go about your daily routine, while working towards better eating habits and choices. No need to worry; this chapter will provide you with hacks that will make the start of your journey simple, and the transition to a better life smoother.

If You Are Working Towards Cutting Calories...

❖ Everyone loves pizza, and the thought of omitting it from your diet can be very daunting. Start slow – *try blotting the oil off the surface of your pizza.* This can actually save you up to 50 calories. When trying to stay within a calorie budget, 50 calories can make all the difference in the world.

Or better yet, try a cauliflower crust pizza — cauliflower is high in fiber and choline, a good source of antioxidants, and may aid in weight loss and it's easy to make *(see recipe in Dinner Recipe section)*.

❖ *Switch your regular bagel for a flat and smaller bagel, eating only half of it. O'Doughs has a great 'thin' bagel.* Bagels contain calories ranging from 300 to 600 easily, add on some toppings such as cream cheese, and that is an additional 50 calories. A great alternative would be to have a corn tortilla with avocado and a splash of salsa, onions and your favorite vegetables.

❖ *Crisp, raw lettuce, arugula or any other greens are highly beneficial in your diet.* These foods contain carotenoids-antioxidants that prevent cells from getting infected and thus work as a shield by blocking cancer in early stages. They are also enriched with high levels fiber, iron, magnesium, potassium, and calcium. Greens have very few carbohydrates, sodium, and cholesterol.

❖ *Try opting for dark meat poultry cuts (chicken thighs, for instance) in place of white cuts (chicken breasts).* Whiter cuts are usually drier, and so we tend to douse them in condiments (ketchup, mayonnaise, mustard, hot sauce, bbq sauce, etc.), which can add empty calories. Darker meats are usually moist and juicy and, contrary to popular belief, have only 10 calories more than white cuts per ounce. Given their moist consistency, it can be easier to avoid condiments and cut out those additional calories. Spice it up a little — black pepper, garlic, fresh ground ginger, and cayenne pepper are awesome additions so that you can avoid higher calorie sauces.

❖ *Dress your pasta, pizza, salad or any other food with balsamic vinegar and olive oil, black pepper or fresh garlic, oregano, instead of cheese.* Spices contain negligible calories, whereas a few tablespoons of Parmesan could easily set you back 50 calories.

❖ *Try avoiding eating salads from fast-food chains or any other place –if you do, order the dressings separately and dress your food yourself.* Fast-food chain salads have many more calories than their burgers, so steer clear of eating them. At restaurants, dress your salads yourself to keep track of the number of condiments that you use.

❖ *Grill, steam or bake your food instead of frying.* You need to add oil or butter when you are frying your food, which adds to the overall calorie count. Cut that out by simply grilling your food, baking it or steaming it. Steaming doesn't need to be plain, try *Steamed Fish with Ginger and Onion* in the 'Dinner Recipe' section. The grill can add a beautiful chargrilled flavor and aroma.

❖ *Eat dark meat fish instead of white meat.* Tuna, cod, mahi-mahi, and such dark meats have fewer calories per ounce when compared to other fish species, such as salmon. Even though salmon contains calories from healthy fats, if your goal is solely to cut calories, then you should make this switch.

Working Towards Increased Protein Intake

❖ *Replace mayonnaise with Greek yogurt.* Greek yogurt constitutes of 10 times more protein as compared to regular mayonnaise, and so is a healthier alternative.

❖ *Substitute your rice with quinoa.* Quinoa is a seed that is high in protein. It is amongst the few rare plant foods that contain all the 9 amino acids. It is also high in fiber, magnesium, B vitamins, iron, potassium, calcium, phosphorus, vitamin E and various beneficial antioxidants.

You can easily replace your oatmeal with quinoa too. An easy quinoa recipe is mentioned in the 'Breakfast Chapter'.

❖ *Add chicken to your salads and meals.* A mere 3 ounces of chicken can supply you with an additional 25 grams of protein.

❖ *Do not waste the liquid that forms on top of your yogurt.* Although that cloudy emission may seem unappealing, it is packed with protein, and so your best option is to mix it back in instead of pouring it out.

❖ There are certain food combinations that supply your body with the 9 necessary amino acids if consumed together, or even separately, within 24 hours. For example, if you are consuming whole-grain cereal, add skim or almond milk to it – which makes a duo of grains and dairy. When eating rice (grains), add dulse or beans to it (legumes). Eat your whole grain bread (grain) with nut butters (legumes). While consuming crackers (grain), use a dip that serves as legumes. A good option can be a black bean dip.

Increasing Your Produce Intake

❖ *Eat your greens cold and raw.* When cooked, greens like spinach or kale will wilt, lose quite a bit of their nutrients and are not as filling once cooked. Opt to eat them raw.

❖ *Combine your cereal or oatmeal with fresh fruit.* Use less cereal (unprocessed like an oatmeal or quinoa) and add fresh fruits, such as strawberries, apples or bananas. These will sweeten your meal naturally and give you a nice, satisfying and energy-packed breakfast.

❖ *Add greens wherever you can.* Big fan of a cheesy grilled sandwich? Just add some lettuce or spinach in there and slowly reduce the amount of cheese so that it complements the greens, instead of the other way around.

❖ *Add vegetables as pizza toppings or to accompany your pasta.* This will be a healthier twist on your favorite dishes, and you will be cutting down calorie consumption without compromising too much.

❖ *Use Avocado as much as you can.* 'Butter' your toast with avocado or guacamole. If it is ripe, it will spread easily and be much more appetizing than a simple butter toast.

❖ *Make use of full-fat salad dressings.* Although this does not actually increase your fresh produce intake, healthy fats (like the ones in olive oil) assist the absorption of the vitamins and nutrients that you get from the produce that you consume.

Try replacing your cereal or oatmeal with smoothie bowls. Here are some quick bowls you might love;

Banana Nut: Blend 1 cup spinach or kale with 1.5 cups of bananas. Add in ¼ cup nuts of your own choice, any milk you want and a dash of cocoa powder.

Berry: Blend 1.5 cup berries with 1 cup kale or spinach, along with the milk of your choice. Add 2 tablespoons of rolled oats and about half a banana.

Green Mango: Blend ½ cup yogurt with 1 cup spinach or kale, and 1.5 cups of mango. Add in 1 cup of water and a little bit of grated ginger (optional).

Pina Colada: Blitz 1 cup coconut water with 1 cup spinach or kale and 1.5 cups of pineapple. Next, mix in 1 tablespoon of chia seeds and shredded coconut.

Green Peach: Blend 1 cup of coconut water with 2 tablespoons of hemp, 1 cup spinach or kale, and 1.5 cups of fresh peaches. Sprinkle ¼ a tablespoon of ground cinnamon if you like.

Cherry Nut: Blend together 1 cup of milk with 2 tablespoons of your choice of nut butter. Mix in 1 cup spinach or kale, and 1.5 cups of cherries.

Working Towards a Decreased Sugar Intake

❖ *Opt for pure dark chocolate in place of chocolate candy.* The same grams of chocolate candy will always contain more sugar than dark chocolate. Replace Mars, Snickers, and Crème Eggs with Pascha, Lindt or other dark chocolates. You may find that even a small square of dark chocolate is enough to keep you satisfied.

❖ *Switch to plain yogurt instead of flavored yogurt.* Flavored yogurt contains at least 15 grams more sugar than plain yogurt.

❖ *Replace dried fruit with fresh fruit.* One cup of raisins contains at least 86 grams of sugar, whereas a cup of grapes has around 15 grams of sugar. While consuming a cup of raisins is unrealistic, it is still better to eat fresh fruit. Dried fruit loses much of the original nutrients and is much higher in sugar.

❖ *Substitute your morning lattes with cappuccinos.* A Starbucks latte contains 17 grams of sugar, whereas the same sized cappuccino contains 10 grams of sugar.

❖ *Opt for unsweetened nut milk in place of your flavored milk.* This will end up helping you cut back on 5 to 15 grams of sugar.

❖ *Choose normal ice cream instead of sorbets.* While choosing sorbets may seem like a better option, on average they contain 12 more grams of sugar than conventional ice cream.

❖ *Choose marinara instead of ketchup.* The marinara sauce contains only 25 percent of the calories that are found in ketchup.

Many of the condiments that we do not think twice before using are full of sugar. For example, an average strawberry jam contains 24 grams of sugar, a barbecue sauce contains 16 grams, ketchup contains 8 grams, and honey mustard has 4 grams. Salsa dips usually have only 2 grams. On the other hand, mayonnaise, hummus, mustard, and hot sauce largely do not contain sugar. It is important to remember not to take a hardball approach. Let your body have a little sugar, but be in charge of how much.

Cutting Back on Carbs

❖ *Opt for lettuce instead of bread.* When you are making tacos or a sandwich, discard the bread or corn taco shells in favor of lettuce. It helps you get rid more calories and simultaneously reduces the number of carbs. The best part is that it does not taste bad either. Minced meat wrapped in a lettuce shell is a healthy meal choice.

❖ *Substitute cauliflower instead of mashed potatoes.* On average, boiled cauliflower has 27 grams fewer carbs than boiled potatoes. Satisfy your craving without loading on carbs. Add garlic, olive oil and a bit of butter. A tasty cauliflower mash recipe is discussed in the 'Sides Chapter'.

❖ *Consume your protein first when having a meal.* Protein is much more filling than any bread. Eat the meat first, and then if you are still hungry, have vegetables or salad.

❖ *Instead of regular pasta* (like fettuccine), use zucchini spirals. Half a cup of raw pasta has 40 grams of carbs, whereas the same amount of zucchini has only 5 grams.

❖ *Make open-face sandwiches.* If you're having a bread craving, opt for open face. This will help you lower your carb intake without having to give them up entirely.

Miscellaneous Tips and Tricks

❖ When baking, try substituting butter, margarine or oil with nut and seed butters, such as almond butter. The calorie count remains the same usually, but nut and seed butters add fiber, good fats and anti-oxidants to your food. A little extra water may be needed for certain recipes, but mostly this switch will work perfectly. (If using almond butter choose organic almond butter as this is one of the crops that use more pesticides than any other crop).

❖ For a dairy-free indulgence, try making whipped cream out of coconut cream. This is a better option than normal whipped cream.

❖ When making tomato sauce for your pasta, incorporate guacamole, avocado, Greek yogurt or coconut milk into it. This will reduce the cream in, which means it will reduce calories, and it will also cut down on the saturated fats.

❖ Apart from using vinegar and water to clean non-organic food, you can use baking soda, lemon juice, water, and vinegar in combination to remove any pesticides.

❖ Try making a soup with pureed vegetables. This will be a much healthier approach and will clean your body from the inside.

❖ If you are addicted to artificial juices, try cutting down by either making fresh juices at home without any additional sweetener or drink fresh fruit infused water. Simply leave a few slices of your favorite fruit in a filled water bottle overnight. My current favorite fresh juice is celery, apple, carrot and lemon.

Unhealthy Item	Healthy Alternative	Fact
Rice	Quinoa	Quinoa has 100% more fiber and 150% more protein than rice.
Mayo	Mustard	Mayo has a lot of saturated fat in it and is high in sugar. Mustard, on the other hand, has neither.
Soda	Tea	Soda contains approximately 8 tsp. of sugar. A healthier option would be tea, which has no sugar and contains healthy antioxidants

Vegetable oil	Coconut oil	Oil in coconut fat contains triglycerides, which help in weight loss.
Sour cream	Greek yogurt	As compared to Sour Cream, Greek yogurt has 3 times more protein and 2 times fewer calories.
Croutons	Almonds	Almonds have three times more fiber and 2 times more protein than croutons It is also just a 1/3 of the carbs.
Potato chips	Popcorn	Popcorn contains nine times less saturated fat and has 1/3 fewer calories than potato chips.
Flour	Coconut flour	Coconut flour contains 11 times the fiber of regular flour and has fewer carbs.
Sugar	Stevia	Stevia has zero sugar, carbs and calories.
Lettuce	Romaine	Romaine has 4 times the vitamin K and 17 times the Vitamin A of Iceberg lettuce.
Bread crumbs	Chia seeds	Chia Seeds is a great alternative to Bread Crumbs because it has 35 times less sodium, 2 times more protein, and 19 times more fiber.
Sports drink	Coconut water	As compared to sports drinks, coconut water has half the sugar of it and 16 times the potassium.

Milk	Almond milk	Almond milk has 6 times fewer calories per glass serving compared to the regular milk.
Peanut butter	Almond butter	Almond butter is free from hydrogenated oils and extra sugars.
Salt	Himalayan crystal salt	Himalayan salt is more natural and is not as harmful as conventional salt.
Chocolate chips	Cacao nibs	Cacao nibs are sugar-free and have 5 times more fiber than normal chocolate chips.

General Guidelines

One of the biggest food tricks is knowing that the key to serving sizes is your hand. First, make sure to compare your hand to a measuring cup. Your fist is usually the size of 1 cup. ½ cup of cooked pasta/rice/vegetables and fruit and 1 cup of raw leafy greens is usually 1 serving. This will help you if you are maintaining a chart.

The palm of your hand is equal to 3 ounces of meat. 2 servings (6 ounces) of any protein (fish, poultry, red meat) should be included in your everyday diet according to nutrition guidelines, unless you are following a specific diet. Your thumb is equal to about 1 ounce of cheese. It is recommended that you have at least 2-3 servings from the dairy group (nutrition pyramid). The tip of your thumb is about the same size as one teaspoon, and your entire thumb is about one tablespoon. It is better if you keep the condiments or butter under one tablespoon a day. While you are snacking, you often do not measure how much you eat. However, it is best to keep in mind that 1 handful is equal to 1 ounce of candies or nuts, when it comes to chips, 2 handfuls are equal to 1 ounce.

Hydration is another vital part of good health. Being dehydrated can make you feel hungry as your body is tricked into believing it needs more food instead of water. Start carrying a water bottle with you that you can refill during the day. If you are exercising and losing a lot of water, you will have to drink more water to compensate for it.

The Institute of Medicine recommends that men drink about 13 cups and women drink about 9 cups of water per day. Or think of it in terms of half to one ounce of water for each pound that you weigh. Stockpile on healthy snacks. Do not go out without any snacks in case of midday hunger strikes, which often leads you to make unhealthy choices. If you have a fridge at work, stock it up on Greek yogurt and boiled eggs so that you can have plenty of protein in the afternoon. Fill your office drawer or purse with nuts, nut butters, bananas, or apples, to make sure you can consume a healthy snack when you are hungry. Pick a day or night during the week where you plan your meals for the week ahead. You can prepare several meals at a time, and you will be probably glad you did once you are running late and can grab a meal that is already prepared on your way out the door. You can even separate snacks into portion-controlled bags. Choosing healthy vegetables for your meals is the most nutrient-dense option. Meal planning is the best way to ensure that you do not splurge at the last minute by giving in to your cravings. Keep your diet simple. Eat lots of vegetables, mostly plants with lots of variety and color. Balance your meals by incorporating lots of proteins into it, such as beans, tofu, fish, and lean meat.

You should even corporate items with complex carbs, such as sweet potato, butternut squash, beets, and brown rice. There are some fats that are healthy for the body, such as olive oil, seeds, nuts, and avocado. Keep away from processed junk food, and the best way to do that is to not bring it to your house or kitchen. This will ensure that you do not get tempted.

Chapter 5
Breakfast Recipes

You might have heard this a lot that a healthy breakfast is the key to start a good day. In this chapter, we will give you an insight into what goes behind making breakfast the most important meal of the entire day. A healthy breakfast not only lets you perform better on the job, but it also supports our overall well-being. It may not be easy to prepare a healthy breakfast in the morning, but having a healthy dish or two really makes the difference. Breakfast means to break the fast. Since your body does not consume anything after dinner, your body is starved.

Breakfast provides your body with fuel. Nutritionists advise consuming breakfast with 20-35% of your daily calorie intake. Your body needs nutrients such as calcium, fiber, vitamins, and carbohydrates in the morning since it is hard to attain them later in the day as well as to get more energy as the body functions throughout the day. A healthy breakfast restores your glucose levels. Glucose is essential for your brain to function. Breakfast is also good for your waistline. Research has shown that those who eat breakfast are less likely to gain weight. Skipping breakfast may lead you to gain weight due to the consumption of high sugar and fatty snack by mid-day. A healthy breakfast will not only improve your performance in school or work but also contribute to your skin. Eggs, lean protein, watermelon, cantaloupe and mango are essential to a healthy breakfast. These foods contain tons of vitamins A and D. These vitamins contribute to maintaining healthy skin. The following are some healthy recipes that are easy for your fast-paced mornings.

Trail Mix Overnight Oats
Serves 1
Calories: 257, Protein: 14g, Total Fat: 11g, Carbohydrates: 33g, Fiber: 5g

Ingredients:
- ❖ ½ cup rolled oats (gluten-free)
- ❖ ¾ cup of water
- ❖ 1 tbsp. dried cranberries
- ❖ 1 tbsp. sunflower seeds and 1tbsp. pumpkin seeds *or*1-2 tbsp. chopped almonds
- ❖ Cinnamon to taste
- ❖ Salt to taste
- ❖ 1 tsp. maple syrup (optional)

Directions:
- ❖ Mix your oats, water, dried cranberries and cinnamon in a bowl or a jar and let it sit overnight in the refrigerator.
- ❖ Add sunflower seeds, pumpkin seeds or almonds, cinnamon and maple syrup in the morning.
- ❖ Your breakfast is ready.

Yogurt Parfait

Serves 1
Calories: 360, Protein: 25g, Total Fat: 14g, Carbohydrates: 42g, Fiber: 8g

Ingredients:
- ❖ 1 cup of full-fat plain Greek Yogurt
- ❖ 1cup of berries or any fruit of your choice
- ❖ ¼ cup of gluten-free granola

Directions:
- ❖ Just add all these ingredients into the bowl, give it a good mix, and enjoy!

Spinach Egg Bake

Serves 4-6
Calories: 206, Protein: 15g, Total Fat: 12g, Carbohydrates: 9g, Fiber: 2g

Ingredients:
- ❖ 1 tbsp. of olive oil
- ❖ 1 small onion (diced)

- ❖ 1 cup chopped spinach
- ❖ 2 garlic scapes (cut into ½ inch pieces)
- ❖ 6 large beaten eggs
- ❖ 1 cup chopped cherry tomatoes
- ❖ ½ cup of cheddar cheese
- ❖ ½ tsp. salt
- ❖ Dash of pepper

Directions:
- ❖ Pre-heat oven to 350°F.
- ❖ Heat olive oil in a cast-iron skillet. You can even use the non-stick pan depending on the availability of resources. But preferably, I would recommend a cast-iron skillet as it is more convenient. Add the diced onion and cook until the onion begins to soften and translucent (about 3 minutes).
- ❖ Add spinach and cook for somewhere around 2 ½ minutes by periodically covering and uncovering it with the lid until the spinach has softened. You will notice the decrease in the volume of the spinach as it softens.
- ❖ Add garlic scapes and cook for 1 minute.
- ❖ Using a whisk, add 6 eggs to a bowl and beat the eggs until they are well mixed. Add chopped cherry tomatoes, salt, and pepper as per your taste.
- ❖ If you're using a cast-iron skillet, add the egg mixture to the skillet and then add your desired topping of any choice of cheese. Or, transfer spinach and egg mixture and top it with cheese to a 9" non-stick pan and bake for the next 35 minutes.

Overnight Breakfast in Bed

Serves 1
Calories: 347, Protein: 27g, Total Fat: 29g,
Carbohydrates: 7g, Fiber: 1g

Ingredients:

- ❖ 2 eggs
- ❖ ¼ cup finely diced red pepper
- ❖ 1 tbsp. shallots
- ❖ 2 tbsp. shredded cheddar cheese
- ❖ 1 slice of crispy bacon (alternatively you can use 1-ounce ham or Canadian bacon)
- ❖ 3 tbsp. salsa
- ❖ Salt and pepper to taste

Preparation:

- ❖ Grease a 7ounce ramekin. Add 3 tbsp. salsa to the bottom of the ramekin. In a bowl, whisk eggs, red pepper, shallots and half of the cheese. Crumble ½ slice of crispy bacon into the egg mixture. Add mixture into ramekin and top with remaining bacon and cheese.
- ❖ Refrigerate it overnight.
- ❖ Preheat oven to 350°F. Bake for 18-22 minutes.

Mushroom & Basil Crustless Quiche

Serves 6-8
Calories: 278, Protein: 12g, Total Fat: 18g, Carbohydrates: 5g, Fiber: 1g

Ingredients:
- ❖ 2 tbsp. olive oil
- ❖ 1 package dried chanterelle mushrooms
- ❖ 1 portobello mushroom (gills removed and chopped into ½ inch squares)
- ❖ 8 ounces of sliced white mushrooms (preferably without stems)
- ❖ 2 finely chopped garlic cloves
- ❖ 1 sweet onion (chopped in a food processor)
- ❖ a handful of finely chopped basil leaves (stems removed)
- ❖ 8 large eggs
- ❖ 1 tbsp. chopped chives
- ❖ ½ cup shredded gruyere cheese

Directions:
- ❖ Preheat your oven to 350°F.
- ❖ Add a cup of boiling water to the Chanterelle and let it sit for a while.
- ❖ Heat a cast-iron skillet or a nonstick pan. Add olive oil.
- ❖ When the oil is heated, add your chopped onions and cook for the next 3-5 minutes, occasionally stirring, until the onion changes its color to slightly translucent.
- ❖ Add garlic cloves and cook for one minute.
- ❖ Stir in Portobello mushrooms and cook until softened, approximately 4 minutes.
- ❖ Add white mushrooms and cook for 3-5 minutes.
- ❖ While the white mushrooms are cooking, remove the chanterelle mushrooms from the water. Mince

the chanterelle mushrooms and add them to the mushroom mixture. Cook for one minute more and then set aside the mushroom and onion mixture.
* Whisk the eggs in a medium-sized bowl and add basil, chives and black pepper to it.
* Line an 8"x8" square pan with parchment paper.
* Pour in the mushroom mixture followed by the egg mixture. Top with shredded cheese.
* Bake for 25-35 minutes.

Homemade Muesli with Oats, Dates & Berries

Serves 4
Calories: 195, Protein: 3g, Total Fat: 4g, Carbohydrates: 41g, Fiber: 7g

Ingredients:
* ½ cup gluten-free oats
* 12 pecans broken into pieces
* 6 pitted dates, cut into pieces
* 1 cup gluten-free rice crisps
* 4 packets of bio yogurt (3 ½ ounces each)
* 2 cups mixed berries (raspberries, strawberries, and blueberries)
* Ground cinnamon (optional)

Directions:
* Fry the oats in a frying pan and heat gently until it starts to toast. Add in the pecans to warm. Transfer to a large bowl and toss to let it cool quickly.

* ❖ Add in the dates and rice crisps in the bowl. Mix it well until it is combined thoroughly.
* ❖ Serve it with yogurt as a topping and add the berries on top. Sprinkle some cinnamon to taste.

Blueberry Muffins

Makes 12
Calories: 190, Protein: 4.5g, Total Fat: 7g, Carbohydrates: 29g, Fiber: 2.6g

Ingredients:
* ❖ 2 eggs, large
* ❖ ½ cup Greek yogurt
* ❖ 3 tbsp. rapeseed oil
* ❖ ¾ cup apple sauce
* ❖ 1 whole banana of medium-size (mashed)
* ❖ 4 tbsp. of regular honey
* ❖ ½ tsp. vanilla extract
* ❖ 1 ½ cups gluten-free cake flour
* ❖ ½ cup gluten-free rolled oats
* ❖ 2 tsp. gluten-free baking powder
* ❖ 1 ½ tsp. baking soda
* ❖ 1 ½ tsp. cinnamon
* ❖ ½ cup blueberries
* ❖ 2 tbsp. of mix seeds (chia, flax, pumpkin, sesame). You can substitute any if you want to.
* ❖ Pinch of salt

Directions:
* ❖ First of all, preheat your oven to 350°F.

❖ Line a muffin tray with muffin cases (muffin paper cups).
❖ In a jug, mix all your wet ingredients; the eggs, yogurt, oil, apple sauce, banana, honey, and vanilla.
❖ In a large bowl, mix in the dry ingredients, including flour, oats, baking powder, baking soda, cinnamon, and blueberries. Don't add your seeds at this step. Now add a pinch of salt and give it a good mix.
❖ Pour the mixture of wet ingredients into the dry and mix until you get a smooth batter. Make sure you don't overmix it as it will make your muffins dense and heavy. Just mix it until all the ingredients are well incorporated.
❖ Now scoop the batter in the muffin tray and sprinkle over your leftover oats and seeds.
❖ Bake the muffins for 25-30 minutes until they turn gold in color and have risen or for better validation, perform a toothpick test. If the toothpick comes out clean, you are good to go. Remove the tray from the oven and let cool on a cooling rack.

Croque Monsieur

Serves 4
Calories: 466, Protein: 29g, Total Fat: 26g,
Carbohydrates: 27g, Fiber: 4g

Ingredients:
❖ 8 slices of gluten-free bread
❖ 1 tbsp. softened butter
❖ 2 cups Emmental cheese

- ❖ 8 Slices ham
- ❖ ¼ cup parmesan cheese
- ❖ ¼ cup cheddar cheese
- ❖ Fresh chives (optional)

Béchamel Sauce:
- ❖ 3-4 tbsp. of softened butter.
- ❖ 3 tbsp. gluten-free flour
- ❖ 2 cups of low fat skimmed milk (or soy if you prefer)
- ❖ 1 tbsp. dry mustard powder (optional)
- ❖ ½ tsp. of onion powder
- ❖ A pinch of salt or as per your taste.
- ❖ Black pepper
- ❖ A pinch of paprika (optional)

Directions:
- ❖ Preheat oven to broil.
- ❖ Butter one side of the bread and assemble the sandwiches (butter will be on the outside of the bread) — layer ¼ cup of Emmental cheese, one slice of ham, ¼ cup of Emmental cheese. Having cheese on both sides of the bread will help the sandwich stay together. Grill the sandwiches to desired crispness and then place all of them onto an oven tray and set aside. For a lighter version, omit the top slice of bread and grill the single slice with ¼ cup of Emmental and one slice of ham but do not flip the bread.

❖ To make the béchamel sauce, add the butter to a pot and heat it at medium to high heat.

❖ As soon as your butter melts down, sift in the flour and add it to the pot, constantly stirring with a whisk to avoid making any lumps. Do not allow the mixture to burn or stick to the bottom of the pot.

❖ Add the milk, and continue to stir and allow the sauce to gradually thicken. Once the mixture boils, you should have reached the desired thickness. Now add your onion powder and salt to the mixture.

❖ Pop in the parmesan cheese and let it melt and get incorporated completely into the sauce. Remove the pan from the heat and let it sit, stirring slowly.

❖ Top sandwiches with ¼ cup of béchamel sauce (or more if you like)

❖ Sprinkle top with shredded cheese and paprika.

❖ Place the assembled sandwiches in the oven and broil until the cheese bubbles (about 5 minutes).

❖ Top with chives - Serve hot.

Cinnamon Crepes with Nut Butter & Dark Chocolate

Serves 2-3
Calories: 302, Protein: 8g, Total Fat: 16g, Carbohydrates: 39g, Fiber: 11g

Ingredients:
❖ ½ cup gluten-free bread flour (do not use bean flour)

❖ 1 tsp. ground cinnamon or cinnamon powder.

❖ ½ tsp. baking powder (gluten-free)

- ❖ 1 egg
- ❖ ¾ cup skim milk
- ❖ 1 tsp. rapeseed oil
- ❖ 2 tbsp. almond nut butter
- ❖ 1 ounce chopped dark chocolate
- ❖ ¾ fresh fruit (optional)
- ❖ 1 tsp. maple syrup (optional)

Directions:

- ❖ Mix your dry ingredients in a separate bowl and your wet ingredients (egg and milk) in another.
- ❖ Now pour the wet mixture into the dry ingredients and whisk until you have a smooth batter. The batter should be lump-free and neither too thick nor too runny. Add more milk; a tablespoon at a time in order to reach desired consistency if the batter is too thick.
- ❖ Place a non-stick pan over the stove and brush it with butter or oil. Now add a small amount of your prepared batter to the pan and give it a good twirl, in order to spread the batter equally throughout the pan, forming a thin layer.
- ❖ As soon as you observe the edges turning brown, flip over the crepe and let it cook for another minute on low heat.
- ❖ Place your crepe on the plate and serve it with nut butter and chocolate. Optional fruit ideas are banana, raspberries, and blueberries.

Banana Peanut Butter Chia Seed Pudding

Serves 2
Calories: 324, Protein: 14g, Total Fat: 11g, Carbohydrates:
41g, Fiber: 6g

Ingredients:
- ❖ 2 ripe bananas
- ❖ 1 ½ cup skim milk
- ❖ 2 tbsp. all-natural creamy peanut butter
- ❖ 3 tbsp. of chia seeds.

Directions:
- ❖ In a blender, mix the banana, milk, and peanut butter. Pour out the mixture in a bowl and mix in the chia seeds. Cover the bowl with the cling film and refrigerate it for the next 4 hours or preferably overnight.
- ❖ Stir the mixture before serving.

Breakfast Quinoa

Serves 2
Calories: 450, Protein: 20g, Total Fat: 8g, Carbohydrates:
36g, Fiber: 6g

Ingredients:
- ❖ 2 cups of low-fat milk (or soy if you prefer)
- ❖ 1 cup rinsed quinoa
- ❖ 2 tbsp. light brown sugar
- ❖ 1/8 tsp. ground cinnamon

Directions:
- ❖ In a saucepan, heat the milk and bring it to the simmer point.
- ❖ Now add in the quinoa and bring the milk to a boil.
- ❖ Reduce the heat to low and let simmer, covered. Cook until ¾ of the milk is absorbed. Approx. 15 minutes.
- ❖ Stir in the sugar and cinnamon and keep the heat on.
- ❖ Cook until all the milk is absorbed. About 8 minutes more. Serve with additional milk, sugar, cinnamon and your favorite fresh fruit.

Chapter 6
Lunch Recipes

We have heard a lot of times that breakfast is the most important meal of the day. It energizes you and provides you with the right amount of nutrition for the entire day ahead. However, when it comes to the stressful professional life, lunch becomes the most important meal of the day. In a survey done on professionals, almost half of the people felt that their productivity levels dropped around 3 pm in the afternoon due to not having lunch.

The question is, why do we skip lunch? Many people said the workload would not let them have lunch. Students said that they mostly avoided having lunch in the cafeteria, and some skipped lunch to participate in extracurricular activities.

What happens when we skip lunch? If you skip lunch, you tend to overeat in your next meal. This practice will make it hard for you to have a proper eating routine. In the race to lose weight, if you are skipping lunch, you are on the wrong track. According to a study, people who skipped meals were seen to gain more weight more as compared to the people who consumed adequate meals throughout the day. Skipping lunch causes you to eat more, or it turns you towards foods with poor nutrition like junk food.

Eating healthy foods for lunch will help in maintaining your metabolism and will keep your body healthy. It is best to combine carbohydrates with lean protein to form a source of long-lasting energy. For example, non-fat yogurt and granola, lean turkey on whole-grain bread, or just cottage cheese with fruits. An ideal lunch is a balance of grains, vegetables, fruits, lean proteins, and dairy.

Below are some lunch recipes that will help revitalize you for the day ahead:

5 Minute Greek Salad
Serves 3
Calories 253, Protein 0.3g, Total Fat 28.3g,
Carbohydrates 1.7g, Fiber 0.8g

Ingredients:
- ❖ 1 English cucumber, diced
- ❖ 10 cherry tomatoes, diced
- ❖ ¼ cup red onion
- ❖ 1 green pepper, diced
- ❖ 1 red pepper, diced

❖ 12 black olives
❖ 1 tbsp. feta cheese

For the Dressing:
❖ 6 tbsp. of olive oil
❖ ¼ cup red wine vinegar
❖ 1 tbsp. fresh lemon juice
❖ 1 garlic clove, minced
❖ 1 tsp. Dijon mustard
❖ 1 tbsp. fresh chopped oregano
❖ Salt and Pepper

Directions:
❖ Toss the chopped vegetables in a separate big bowl.
❖ Place all dressing ingredients in a mason jar and shake vigorously until mixed well. Add in the oregano after the dressing is ready.
❖ Top with black olives and crumbled feta and enjoy!

Apple Cider Vinegar Dressing with Mixed Greens

Serves 4
Calories 70, Protein 0.4g, Total Fat 6g, Carbohydrates 4g, Fiber 0g

Ingredients:
❖ 1 garlic clove, minced
❖ 1 tbsp. Dijon Mustard
❖ ¼ cup raw apple cider vinegar
❖ 2 tbsp. fresh lemon juice

- ❖ 1-2 tbsp. raw honey
- ❖ 1/3 cup extra-virgin olive oil
- ❖ Salt and Pepper

Directions:
- ❖ Combine all the ingredients into a mason jar or any shaker and shake vigorously until all the ingredients are blended.
- ❖ Adjust the flavor as per taste.
- ❖ Toss with your favorite mixed greens.

Rainbow Ranch Veggie Pinwheels

Serves 4
Calories 304, Protein 13g, Total Fat 17g, Carbohydrates 23g, Fiber 2g

Ingredients:
- ❖ 4 large tortillas (gluten-free)
- ❖ 1 avocado
- ❖ ½ cup sliced bell peppers
- ❖ ½ cup thinly sliced carrot strips
- ❖ ½ cup thinly sliced yellow bell pepper strips
- ❖ ½ cup of mixed greens
- ❖ ½ cup of finely chopped purple cabbage

Dressing:
- ❖ ½ cup mayonnaise
- ❖ ½ cup sour cream
- ❖ 1 teaspoon dried dill weed
- ❖ 1 teaspoon fresh parsley

- ❖ 1 teaspoon fresh chives
- ❖ ¼ teaspoon onion powder
- ❖ ½ teaspoon garlic powder
- ❖ ¼ teaspoon fine sea salt
- ❖ Dash of cayenne (optional)

Directions:
- ❖ Add the mayonnaise, sour cream, dill, parsley, chives, onion powder, garlic powder, salt, and cayenne (optional) and blend well.
- ❖ Add equal amounts of all the cut vegetables and avocado in a straight line and top it with the dressing.
- ❖ Roll the tortilla tightly into a wrap.
- ❖ Cut crosswise into pinwheels and serve.

Chicken Salad with Ginger-Sesame Dressing

Serves 6
Calories 294, Protein 15g, Total Fat 14g, Carbohydrates 2g, Fiber 4g
Ingredients:
For the salad
- ❖ 2 chicken breasts, cooked and cut in slices (for a pescatarian option use 12-16 cooked shrimp)
- ❖ 4 cups mixed greens
- ❖ ¼ cup radicchio (optional)
- ❖ 1 whole diced red bell pepper
- ❖ ½ small red onion, diced
- ❖ 2 tbsp. fresh cilantro, chopped

- ❖ ½ cup pomegranate
- ❖ ½ cup slivered almonds

For the dressing (can also be used as a marinade)
- ❖ 2 tbsp. of olive oil
- ❖ 3 ½ tbsp. lime juice
- ❖ 2 tsp. soy sauce
- ❖ 1 tsp. of minced ginger
- ❖ 2 ½ tsp. sesame oil
- ❖ 2 garlic cloves, minced
- ❖ 1/8 tsp. red pepper flakes

Directions:
- ❖ Add mixed greens to a bowl and add bell pepper and cilantro. Combine well.
- ❖ In a separate bowl, mix together all the ingredients for the dressing. Now give it a good mix and then pour the dressing over the salad.
- ❖ Stir to distribute it evenly.
- ❖ Season with salt and pepper.
- ❖ Slice chicken and serve over top.
- ❖ Top with almonds and pomegranate and serve chilled or at room temp.

Directions For the Chicken:
- ❖ Preheat oven to 350°F.
- ❖ There are a few options:
- ❖ Sprinkle with onion powder, crushed garlic, and oregano.

Or

❖ Marinade chicken overnight in:
❖ ¾ cup olive oil (extra virgin)
❖ ¼ cup apple cider vinegar
❖ 5 garlic cloves (crushed)
❖ 2 tbsp. of Worcestershire sauce
❖ 1 tbsp. lemon juice
❖ ½ tsp. salt
❖ ½ tsp. black pepper
❖ Bake for the 30 minutes or until the juices run clear.

Kale Quinoa Salad with Feta and a Honey-Lemon Vinaigrette

Serves 4
Calories 298, Protein 13g, Total Fat 21g, Carbohydrates 12g, Fiber 10g

Ingredients
Salad
❖ 1 cup uncooked quinoa
❖ 4 cups kale, washed and stems removed, cut into small ribbons
❖ 1/3 cup feta cheese, crumbled
❖ 1 cup chickpeas
❖ 2 tbsp. red onion, diced
❖ 1 avocado, cubed

Vinaigrette
❖ 3 tbsp. of extra virgin olive oil
❖ 3 tbsp. apple cider vinegar

- ❖ 1 tsp. fresh lemon juice
- ❖ 2 tsp. honey
- ❖ ½ tsp. lemon zest
- ❖ 2 tbsp. olive oil

Directions
- ❖ Cook quinoa as per instructions given on the package. Set aside to cool.
- ❖ In a bowl, whisk together the ingredients to make the vinaigrette.
- ❖ Add kale in the vinaigrette and toss well. Make sure that the kale is coated with the vinaigrette.
- ❖ Add in the cooked quinoa when it is cooled.
- ❖ Toss in the rest of the salad ingredients and mix well.
- ❖ Add the avocado on top right before serving.

Caprese Chicken Salad
Serves 4
Calories 364, Protein 22g, Total Fat 6g, Carbohydrates 3g, Fiber 3g

Ingredients
Salad
- ❖ ¾ cup quinoa, uncooked
- ❖ 1 tbsp. balsamic vinegar
- ❖ 1 tbsp. olive oil
- ❖ ¼ tsp. crushed rosemary
- ❖ 2 large skinless, boneless chicken breasts
- ❖ 3 cups cherry tomatoes cut in halves

❖ 1 cup baby bocconcini
❖ 1 cup of basil leaves, stems removed

Balsamic Vinaigrette
❖ 3 tbsp. balsamic vinegar
❖ 3 tbsp. olive oil
❖ 1 tbsp. maple syrup
❖ ¼ tsp. Dijon mustard
❖ Salt and pepper to taste

Directions
❖ Cook quinoa as per package instructions. Let cool.
❖ Preheat your oven to 425°F.
❖ Season the chicken with balsamic vinegar, rosemary, salt, pepper, and olive oil.
❖ Bake for 22-28 minutes until the chicken is cooked thoroughly and juices run clear.
❖ Rest the chicken before cutting into cubes.
❖ In a bowl, mix the vinaigrette ingredients together.
❖ In a bigger bowl, toss all the salad ingredients along with the chicken. Mix well.
❖ Drizzle the vinaigrette over the salad and mix well.

Ginger Edamame Quinoa
Serves 4
Calories 275, Protein 16.7g, Total Fat 8.8g, Carbohydrates 34.9g, Fiber 7.6g

Ingredients

- ❖ 2 cups of water
- ❖ 1 cup of quinoa
- ❖ 2 tbsp. extra virgin olive oil
- ❖ 1 onion, diced
- ❖ 1 bell pepper, diced
- ❖ 2 cups of broccoli cut in medium bite-size chunks
- ❖ 1 tsp. freshly grated ginger
- ❖ 1 garlic clove crushed
- ❖ 1 can (14 oz.) black beans (organic in a BPA free can)
- ❖ 3 tbsp. of gluten-free soy sauce
- ❖ 1 cup edamame
- ❖ 2 cups of diced protein of your choice (chicken, beef, pork, shrimp or tofu), cooked

Directions

- ❖ Boil the quinoa in 2 cups of water in a saucepan over the stove. Cover the lid, and let it simmer for the next 10-12 minutes.
- ❖ Remove the saucepan from the heat and keep covered for 6 minutes. Fluff the quinoa with a fork and set it aside.
- ❖ Heat a large saucepan heat the oil, and onion and cook for 4 minutes.
- ❖ Add garlic and ginger and cook for the next 3 minutes.
- ❖ Add broccoli and cook for another 2 minutes — until the broccoli is tender from the inside but still have the outer crisp (al dente).

❖ Toss in the bell pepper, protein, black beans, edamame, and soy sauce.
❖ Stir in the fluffed quinoa and serve it hot.

Crock-pot Chicken Tetrazzini
Serves 4-6
Calories 285, Protein 37.3g, Total Fat 9.4g, Carbohydrates 6.6g, Fiber 0.7g

Ingredients

❖ 6 boneless skinless chicken breasts or 12 boneless skinless chicken thighs (2 ½ to 3 lbs.)
❖ 3/4 cup of water
❖ 3/4 cup white wine
❖ 1 medium onion, coarsely chopped
❖ 1 tsp. salt
❖ ¼ tsp. thyme
❖ ¼ tsp. pepper
❖ 2 tbsp. finely chopped parsley
❖ 1 bulb of garlic (about 10 whole cloves)

Thickening agent
❖ ¼ cup of water
❖ 2 tbsp. corn starch

Directions
❖ In a crockpot combine chicken, water, wine, onion, salt, thyme salt, pepper, parsley, and garlic cloves.

Cover the lid and let it cook for a minimum of 10 – 12 minutes.

❖ Using two forks, shred the chicken into fine thin threads. Strain the broth into a saucepan saving the onion and garlic.

❖ Add the garlic and onions in a food processor to make a puree. Set aside

❖ Bring broth to a boil. Mix thickening agent (¼ cup of water and 2 tbsp. cornstarch). When broth is boiling, slowly add thickening agents while whisking constantly. You may wish to add a pinch of thyme to enhance the flavor. Stir in the garlic and onion puree. Add the chicken back in and stir.

❖ Serve over rice or gluten-free pasta.

Chicken & Kale Lasagna
Serves 4-6
Calories 420, Protein 28g,
Total Fat 18g, Carbohydrates 31g, Fiber 2g

Ingredients
❖ 2 cups Béchamel sauce (recipe below)
❖ 2 lbs. cooked chicken breasts chopped into ½ inch cubes
❖ 1 cup of frozen kale (chopped)
❖ 2 cloves of garlic (crushed)
❖ 1 small onion, diced
❖ Salt and pepper to taste
❖ 1 (8 oz.) tub cottage cheese
❖ 2 cups shredded cheddar and mozzarella cheese mixture

❖ Gluten-free lasagna noodles

For the Béchamel sauce:
❖ 2 cups of milk
❖ 4 tbsp. butter
❖ 2 tbsp. of gluten-free, all-purpose flour
❖ ½ cup Parmesan cheese
❖ A pinch of cayenne pepper
❖ A dash of black pepper and salt

Directions
❖ Preheat oven to 350°F F.

To prepare béchamel sauce:
❖ Melt the butter in a saucepan over the medium-low heat. Whisk in the flour and make a runny paste out of it. Avoid letting it turn brown.
❖ Gradually add milk while whisking continuously to avoid any lumps.
❖ Increase the heat to a medium and continue stirring for the next 4 to 5 minutes, until the sauce thickens
❖ Add salt and cayenne pepper.
❖ (You can use the sauce either right away or store it in a lidded jar for the next two days in a refrigerator).
❖ Add cooked chicken, kale, garlic, onion, salt, and pepper to the bechamel sauce and cook on low for 10 minutes.

- ❖ In a rectangular pan, add a layer of the sauce mixture and dollops of cottage cheese (half of the tub)
- ❖ The next layer will be lasagna noodles. Followed by a layer of sauce. Then a layer of the cheese mixture. Next, a layer of lasagna noodles topped with a layer of sauce mix. Finally, top with a layer of shredded cheese.
- ❖ Bake for the 25 to 30 minutes until the cheese melts and turns golden.

Honey Sriracha Glazed Meatballs
Serves 4
Calories 395, Protein 26g,
Total Fat 11g, Carbohydrates 19g, Fiber 1g

Ingredients
For the meatballs
- ❖ 1 lb. lean turkey, ground
- ❖ 1 egg
- ❖ ½ tsp. minced garlic
- ❖ ½ cup sweet onions, diced
- ❖ ¼ cup finely diced red peppers
- ❖ ½ cup gluten-free bread crumbs
- ❖ ½ tsp. salt
- ❖ 2 tbsp. black sesame seeds

For the sauce
- ❖ ¼ cup sriracha
- ❖ 1 ½ tbsp. rice vinegar

- ❖ 1 ½ tbsp. honey
- ❖ 1 ½ tbsp. soy sauce
- ❖ ½ tbsp. grated ginger
- ❖ 2 garlic cloves, minced
- ❖ ½ tsp. sesame oil

Directions
- ❖ Preheat the oven to 375°F.
- ❖ In a large bowl, mix together ground turkey, breadcrumbs, egg, onions, red pepper, garlic, salt, and pepper until well combined. Shape the mixture to make meatballs and place it 1-inch apart on greased baking sheets.
- ❖ Bake the meatballs for 20 to 25 minutes, until browned and cooked. Turn meatballs halfway through cooking.
- ❖ In a saucepan, combine all the ingredients for the sauce and bring to a boil. Whisk continuously. Reduce heat and let simmer for 8 to 10 minutes on medium-low heat until the sauce thickens. Toss in the meatballs.
- ❖ Serve over brown rice and top with sesame seeds.

Wild Mushroom & Cheese Crostini

Serves 4
Calories 276, Protein 27g, Total Fat 8g, Carbohydrates 23g, Fiber 3g

Ingredients:
- ❖ 1 package dried chanterelle mushrooms

❖ 1 cup of warm water
❖ 1 ¼ cups white mushrooms, sliced
❖ 2 portobello diced mushrooms, stems and gills removed
❖ A handful of oyster mushrooms finely chopped
❖ ½ large sweet onion, sliced
❖ 1 tsp. ground thyme
❖ Gluten-free crostini
❖ ½ tsp. oregano
❖ 2 garlic cloves, crushed
❖ ½ cup mayonnaise
❖ ½ cup parmesan cheese

Directions:
❖ Add the chanterelle mushrooms to the warm water and set aside.
❖ Heat oil in a large nonstick skillet, sauté onions until the onions are tender and golden brown, then add one garlic clove and cook for one minute longer.
❖ Add portobello mushrooms and sauté for 4 minutes. Mix in the white mushrooms and sauté for another 3-5 minutes until water has evaporated from the pan.
❖ Remove the chanterelle mushrooms from the water and finely chop. Add chanterelle and oyster mushrooms to the skillet and sauté for another 2-4 minutes. Add in ½ cup of white wine and cook until the wine has evaporated, stirring occasionally.
❖ In a small bowl, combine mayonnaise, oregano, and parmesan cheese. Spread the mixture evenly on the

crostini slices. (Alternatively, you can use feta cheese).

❖ Broil for 3 or 4 minutes until the cheese begins to brown and turn crisp.

❖ Top the crostini with mushroom mixture. Serve warm.

Quick Turkey Taco Lunch Bowls

Serves 4
Calories 387, Protein 23g,
Total Fat 10g, Carbohydrates 42g, Fiber 5g

Ingredients

❖ Romaine hearts

Turkey

❖ ¾ lb. lean turkey, ground
❖ 1 tbsp. extra virgin olive oil
❖ 1 ½ tbsp. chili powder
❖ 1 crushed garlic clove
❖ ½ Spanish onion
❖ ¼ tsp. crushed red pepper flakes
❖ ¼ tsp. dried oregano
❖ ½ tsp. paprika
❖ 1 ½ tsp. ground cumin
❖ ½ tsp. salt

Salsa

❖ 1 jalapeno, minced
❖ 1-pint cherry tomatoes, cut in quarters

❖ Juice of ½ lime
❖ ¼ cup red onion, minced
❖ 1/8 tsp. salt

Directions
❖ Chop the romaine.
❖ Heat the oil in cast iron pan.
❖ Combine the onion and all of the spices the turkey. Cook for 15 to 20 minutes until cooked through.
❖ In a separate bowl, mix the salsa ingredients and toss.
❖ Serve turkey and salsa over chopped romaine.

Honey Sesame Chicken Lunch Bowls
Serves 4
Calories 445, Protein 33g, Total Fat 11g, Carbohydrates 56g, Fiber 3g

Ingredients
❖ ¾ cup uncooked rice
❖ 3 cups broccoli, chopped to small pieces
❖ 3 cups green beans, cut into 1-inch pieces
❖ 1 tbsp. of extra virgin olive oil
❖ 2 large chicken breasts, diced
❖ 1 clove garlic (crushed)
❖ Red pepper flakes
❖ Black sesame seeds for the topping
❖ Salt and pepper to taste

Honey Sesame Sauce
- ❖ ¼ cup soy sauce
- ❖ 1 tbsp. sesame oil
- ❖ ¼ cup chicken stock
- ❖ ¼ cup honey
- ❖ 1 tsp. cornstarch
- ❖ ½ tsp. red pepper flakes

Directions
- ❖ Mix all the ingredients of the honey sesame sauce in a bowl and set aside.
- ❖ Cook the rice according to the package instructions.
- ❖ For the chicken heat olive oil in a large pan over medium-high heat.
- ❖ Season the chicken with garlic, salt, black pepper, and red pepper flakes. Cook for 7 minutes per side until cooked through (15 to 25 minutes).
- ❖ Add in the broccoli and green beans. Cook for 2 to 3 minutes until color changes to bright green and the beans become tender.
- ❖ Pour the sauce in the pan and simmer it for another 2 minutes until it thickens.
- ❖ To serve, place rice on a plate and add the chicken on top, garnish with sesame seeds.

Butternut Squash and White Bean Soup

Serves 4 - 6
Calories 250, Protein 7g, Total Fat 12.5g, Carbohydrates:
31g, Fiber 4g

Ingredients
- ❖ 1 large butternut squash
- ❖ 1 chopped onion
- ❖ 2 tbsp. of extra virgin olive oil.
- ❖ The 1-inch ginger piece, grated
- ❖ 2 garlic cloves (finely chopped)
- ❖ 6 cups of vegetable broth, low sodium
- ❖ 6 sprigs fresh thyme
- ❖ 1 bay leaf
- ❖ 1 (14oz.) can of white beans, rinsed and drained thoroughly
- ❖ 1 can (14 oz.) of chickpeas, drained and rinsed
- ❖ ½ cup red quinoa
- ❖ ¼ cup fresh cilantro, chopped
- ❖ 1 scallion, sliced

Directions
- ❖ Peel and cut the squash to ½ inch pieces.
- ❖ Heat 1 tbsp. of oil in a non-stick pan on medium heat. Add the squash and cook. Stir occasionally for 8 minutes.
- ❖ Heat the remaining oil in a separate pan. Add the onion and cook covered for 6 minutes. Add in the garlic and cook it for another minute or two.

❖ Add broth, thyme, squash, and bring to a boil. With the help of a fork, mash the white beans and add them to the soup. Add in the chickpeas as well.

❖ Cook the quinoa as per the package instructions. When cooked, fluff with the help of a fork. Fold in the cilantro and scallion.

❖ Serve the soup topped with the quinoa mixture.

Korean Pineapple Shrimp Lettuce Wraps

Serves 3
Calories 145, Protein 7.5g,
Total Fat 7g, Carbohydrates 1g, Fiber 0g

Ingredients

❖ ¼ cup of pineapple juice
❖ 1 garlic clove, grated
❖ 1 tbsp. soy sauce
❖ ½ tsp. red pepper flakes
❖ ½ tbsp. grated fresh ginger
❖ ½ tbsp. honey
❖ ½ tbsp. toasted sesame oil
❖ 12 - 18 shrimps
❖ 1 tbsp. of olive oil
❖ Salt
❖ Butter lettuce leaves
❖ Scallions
❖ 1 red bell pepper, sliced thin
❖ 3 carrots, cut into matchsticks
❖ ½ small zucchini, cut into matchsticks

Directions

- ❖ In a medium bowl mix pineapple juice, garlic, soy sauce, red pepper flakes, ginger, honey, and sesame oil.
- ❖ Now add the shrimp into the mixture, cover and refrigerate the marinade for 3 to 4 hours.
- ❖ Take the mixture out of the refrigerator 30 minutes before cooking. Heat a large skillet and add 1 tbsp. extra virgin olive oil.
- ❖ Add the shrimp mixture to the skillet cook for 1 t 5 minutes or until shrimp is cooked.
- ❖ Serve with lettuce leaves, red bell pepper, carrots, zucchini, and scallions.

Salmon with Mango and Lime Salsa

Serves 1
Calories 303, Protein 1g,
Total Fat 0g, Carbohydrates 15g, Fiber 2g

Ingredients

- ❖ 1 (6 oz.) salmon fillet, deboned and skinless
- ❖ 1 tsp. olive oil
- ❖ Salt and pepper to taste

For salsa

- ❖ 1 diced mango
- ❖ Zest and juice of 1 lime
- ❖ ¾ cup diced red bell pepper
- ❖ 2 tbsp. cilantro, chopped
- ❖ 2 thinly sliced scallions

❖ 1 tsp. sriracha or hot sauce (optional)
❖ Salt to taste

Directions
❖ Rub salt and pepper on both sides of salmon fillet.
❖ In a nonstick pan, add 1 tbsp. of olive oil and heat it at medium-high heat.
❖ Add the salmon to the pan and cook for 1 to 2 minutes on both sides until each side turns brown.
❖ Place the salmon on a baking sheet and bake for 8 minutes on 400°F to cook it thoroughly inside out.
❖ In a bowl, mix together cut mangoes, scallions, cilantro, lime juice, lemon zest, sriracha sauce, salt, and red bell peppers.
❖ Serve salmon over jasmine rice and top with the salsa mixture.

Chapter 7
Dinner Recipes

Having a healthy dinner is what satisfies the body after a long hard day at work. A lot of people would agree that going to bed empty stomach is the most unpleasant feeling in the world. You feel drowsy in the morning and the whole day goes lazy. Not having dinner the night before may get your day started in the wrong direction that in turn can also affect your fitness and weight loss journeys. Therefore, if you are further thinking to skip dinner, you might want to think again.

There are a number of benefits to eating dinner. To start with, dinner helps keep your metabolism is running fast. Sitting down to eat is more than just eating. It can improve the way your body functions. When you are worn out at the end of the day your body could be lagging. A healthy and wholesome dinner can enhance your metabolic functions and in turn, it can promote greater success in losing weight. A satisfying meal is the best way to end a long day. You might not have the time to have a proper breakfast and just rush while eating, and you have your lunch under too much pressure. Therefore, dinner is where you want to make up for the missing nutrients during the day. A healthy dinner can help promote brain function, improved digestion and give you proper sleep. Here are a few recipes to help you rejuvenate your body and your overall mood after a long tiring day.

Spicy Curried Lentils (Slow Cooker)
Serves 4 - 6
Calories 168, Protein 9.5g,
Total Fat 4.5g, Carbohydrates 24g, Fiber 10g

Ingredients
- 1 medium shallot, diced
- ½ jalapeno pepper
- ½ can tomato paste
- 3 cloves of garlic
- 2 slices of peeled ginger
- 1 tsp. ground cumin
- 1 tsp. ground coriander
- 1 cup dried brown lentils
- 1 cup of vegetable broth
- 1 ½ cups large cauliflower florets (stems removed)
- ½ tbsp. fresh lime juice
- ½ can coconut milk
- 1 cup of water
- Salt & Pepper
- Steamed rice

Directions

- ❖ In a food processor, toss in your shallot, jalapeno pepper, tomato paste, garlic, ginger, cumin, coriander, salt, pepper, salt, and pepper.
- ❖ Add the mixture to a slow cooker. In the same slow cooker bowl, add the broth, lentils, coconut milk and water. Stir the mixture to combine well. Place the cauliflower on top.
- ❖ Cover and cook on low heat for 4 hours or until the lentils are soft.
- ❖ Lastly, lime juice and add salt to taste.
- ❖ Serve with steamed rice.

Chicken Thighs with Honey Mustard

Serves 5
Calories 230, Protein 30g,
Total Fat 9g, Carbohydrates 6g, Fiber 0g

Ingredients:

- ❖ 3 tbsp. olive oil
- ❖ 1tbsp. honey
- ❖ 2 tbsp. Dijon mustard
- ❖ 4 garlic cloves, finely chopped
- ❖ ½ tsp. ginger paste
- ❖ 2 lbs. skinless boneless chicken thighs
- ❖ Sliced red pepper
- ❖ Salt
- ❖ Pepper

Directions:

- ❖ Preheat the oven to 375°F.
- ❖ Mix in the first five ingredients (honey, mustard, garlic, ginger, and olive oil) in a zip-lock bag.
- ❖ Add salt and pepper to the bag according to your taste buds.
- ❖ Place the chicken in the same bag and seal the bag. Shake the bag and toss the chicken to coat each piece evenly.
- ❖ Refrigerate overnight.
- ❖ When ready to cook, add the chicken to a baking dish. Top with sliced red pepper. Bake the chicken in the oven for 25 minutes.

❖ Flip the chicken and cook it for the next 10 minutes evenly from both sides to ensure the chicken is cooked through.

Chicken with Spinach & Sun-Dried Tomatoes

Serves 4
Calories 335, Protein 33.5g,
Total Fat 21.4g, Carbohydrates 2.9g, Fiber 0.5g

Ingredients:

❖ ½ cup sun-dried tomato paste
❖ 1 lb. skinless, boneless chicken breast cubed (or cubed pacific salmon)
❖ 2 cups of chicken broth (low sodium)
❖ 4 ounces of cream cheese
❖ 1 package (5 oz.) of chopped frozen spinach
❖ ¼ tsp. crushed chili pepper flakes
❖ 3 garlic cloves, minced
❖ ¼ tsp. salt
❖ ¼ tsp. of ground black pepper

Directions:

❖ Heat 1 ½ tsp. of the oil in a large skillet.
❖ Add chicken and cook for 7 minutes on each side.
❖ Add sun-dried tomato paste, garlic, chili pepper, and cook for another 5 minutes.
❖ Now add your chicken broth and cook it for another 6 to 7 minutes.

❖ Mix in the cream cheese and the spinach. Cook until the chicken is cooked and you have a nice creamy sauce.

Salmon with Coconut Cream Tomato Sauce

Serves 4
Calories 301, Protein 30.2g,
Total Fat 17.6g, Carbohydrates 6.9g, Fiber 1.3g

Ingredients:

❖ 1 lb. skinless salmon, cut into 1-inch pieces
❖ 2 tsp. olive oil
❖ 1 small onion, finely chopped
❖ 1 tbsp. minced ginger
❖ 2 cloves garlic, finely chopped
❖ ½ cup drained canned tomatoes, pureed
❖ ½ cup coconut milk
❖ ¼ tsp. cayenne (optional)
❖ 1 cup diced cherry tomatoes
❖ 2 tsp. lemon juice
❖ 2 tbsp. freshly chopped cilantro
❖ Salt and pepper to taste

Directions:

❖ Rub the salt on both sides of the salmon and set aside.
❖ Heat oil in a non-stick skillet. Add onion and garlic and frequently stir until the onions soften. Add ginger and constantly stir for about 20 seconds. Add

pureed tomatoes, coconut milk, and cayenne; simmer uncovered for 5 minutes.

❖ Add cherry tomatoes and simmer for 1 minute. Add salmon and lime, cook on low for about 3-4 minutes or until salmon is cooked. Stir in cilantro.

❖ Serve over brown rice.

Grilled Balsamic Rosemary Flat Iron Steak

Serves 4
Calories 493, Protein 52.7g,
Total Fat 23.1g, Carbohydrates 8.6g, Fiber 0.1g

Ingredients:

❖ 6 cloves minced garlic
❖ ¼ cup extra virgin olive oil
❖ ¼ cup balsamic vinegar
❖ ½ cup dry red wine
❖ 2 tbsp. chopped fresh rosemary
❖ ½ tsp. salt
❖ pinch of black pepper
❖ 1 ¼ lb. flat iron steak

Directions:

❖ In a bowl, add olive oil, balsamic vinegar, red wine along with 1 tbsp. rosemary, salt, and pepper. Give it a good mix until all the ingredients are well incorporated.

❖ Place the steak in a zip-lock bag and pour in your marinade into the bag. Shake the bag to coat the fillet perfectly from each side. Refrigerate your steak overnight to help it absorb the flavors.

❖ Preheat your grill to medium heat.

❖ Place the steak on the grill. Don't throw the residual marinade, we will use it later in the dish.

❖ Cook the steak 3-5 minutes per side or until desired doneness. Remove steak and let rest for 10 minutes. Remember, steak will continue to cook even when resting.

❖ Pour the marinade into a skillet over medium heat. Bring to a boil and let cook until it reduces to half. Stir the remaining rosemary and remove from heat.

❖ After the steak has rested for a minute or two, slice it against the grain into slices half-inch thick.

❖ Drizzle the sauce over the steak.

Marinated Pork Chops
Serves 6
Calories 330, Protein 37.1g,
Total Fat 10.8g, Carbohydrates 20.7g, Fiber 0g

Ingredients:
❖ 6 boneless loin pork chops (1-inch thick)
❖ 12 tablespoons of extra virgin olive oil
❖ 4 tablespoons of apple cider vinegar
❖ 5 crushed garlic cloves
❖ 2 tbsp. Worcestershire sauce
❖ 1 tbsp. lemon juice
❖ 1 tsp. Dijon mustard
❖ A pinch of dried parsley
❖ ½ tsp. salt

❖ A dash of black pepper

Directions:
❖ In a resealable bag, add olive oil, apple cider vinegar, garlic, Worcestershire sauce, lemon juice, Dijon mustard, parsley, salt, and pepper. Add the pork chops to the zip-lock bag.
❖ Toss the chops in the bag, seal, and refrigerate overnight.
❖ Remove pork chops from the marinade. Discard marinade.
❖ Grill the meat over medium-high heat for 5 to 6 minutes until well done from both sides.
❖ Let rest for 5 minutes before serving. Serve with cauliflower mash and steamed broccoli.

Cauliflower Pizza Crust
Serves 3
Calories 155, Protein 2g,
Total Fat 5g, Carbohydrates 24g, Fiber 2g

Ingredients:
❖ 1 medium cauliflower, stalk removed
❖ 2eggs, beaten
❖ 1 clove minced garlic
❖ ½ tsp. oregano
❖ ¾ cup grated cheese (mozzarella, cheddar or Edam)
❖ Salt and Pepper to taste

Directions:

- ❖ Chop the cauliflower into small florets and pulse it into the food processor until finely chopped.
- ❖ Steam in ½ inch of boiling water (covered) until soft. About 7 minutes.
- ❖ Pour out cooked cauliflower onto a clean towel. Make sure to remove all the liquid.
- ❖ Place the cauliflower in a bowl and add egg, oregano, and grated cheese. Mix well until a ball is formed.
- ❖ Place the ball of cauliflower dough onto the center of the pizza stone and press to form a pizza shape.
- ❖ Spray the top with some olive oil and bake at 400°F (180°C) for the next 15 to 20 minutes until it turns golden.
- ❖ Add your desired toppings, cook for 10 to 12 minutes.

Clams Casino

Serves 5
Calories 300, Protein 15g,
Total Fat 15g, Carbohydrates 30g, Fiber 0g

Ingredients:

- ❖ 18 small clams, scrubbed and cleaned well
- ❖ ½ cup of water
- ❖ 2 bay leaves
- ❖ 1 tbsp. of olive oil
- ❖ 2 medium shallots, finely chopped
- ❖ 1 small green bell pepper, chopped
- ❖ 2 tsp. of apple cider vinegar

- ❖ ¾ cup gluten-free breadcrumbs
- ❖ ½ cup grated parmesan cheese
- ❖ 2 tbsp. chopped chives
- ❖ 1tsp. dried oregano
- ❖ ½ tsp. smoked paprika
- ❖ ½ tsp. ground pepper

Directions:

- ❖ Preheat your oven to 450°F.
- ❖ Add the clams, bay leaves and water to a saucepan. Cover the lid and bring it to a boil.
- ❖ Reduce the heat to medium-low and continue to cook until the clams pop open.
- ❖ Drain water from the pan and throw away unopened clams.
- ❖ In a nonstick skillet, heat olive oil over medium heat.
- ❖ Toss in your shallots and bell pepper to the skillet and stir until they are soft.
- ❖ Now take a large bowl and transfer everything into a bowl. Add a splash of vinegar and stir in your breadcrumbs, parmesan, chives spices, and the meat from the clams.
- ❖ Stir everything and stuff the mixture back to the clamshells.
- ❖ Bake for 20 minutes and serve.

Steamed Fish with Ginger and Onion

Serves 4
Calories 317, Protein 40g,
Total Fat 12g, Carbohydrates 12g, Fiber 2g

Ingredients:

- ❖ 4 (5 oz.) fillets of white fish
- ❖ 3.5 lbs. of bok choy
- ❖ 1 tbsp. grated ginger
- ❖ 1 tsp. of rice wine
- ❖ 2 garlic cloves, sliced
- ❖ 2 tbsp. low sodium soy sauce
- ❖ Coriander, chopped
- ❖ Bunch of finely chopped spring onion
- ❖ Brown rice (to serve)
- ❖ 1 lemon, cut into slices
- ❖ 4 parchment bags

Directions:

- ❖ Preheat the oven to 350°F.
- ❖ Divide bok choy into 4 portions and place in parchment bags and place in the refrigerator.
- ❖ Mix the fish, ginger, and garlic in a bowl.
- ❖ Drizzle the soy sauce and rice wine over the fish and season it with salt and pepper.
- ❖ Wrap the bag closed and cook for 20 minutes.
- ❖ Boil some brown rice and squeeze lemon juice over the entire dish before serving.

Meatball Nirvana

Serves 4
Calories 456, Protein 40g,
Total Fat 22g, Carbohydrates 21g, Fiber 2g

Ingredients:

- ❖ 1 lb. organic lean ground beef
- ❖ 1 egg
- ❖ ¾ tsp. crushed red pepper flakes
- ❖ ½ tsp. sea salt
- ❖ 1 dash hot pepper sauce
- ❖ 1 medium-sized onion, diced
- ❖ 1 ½ tbsp. Worcestershire sauce
- ❖ ½ tsp. garlic salt
- ❖ 1 ½ tsp. Italian seasoning
- ❖ ¼ grated parmesan cheese
- ❖ ¾ tsp. dried oregano
- ❖ ½ cup gluten-free breadcrumbs, seasoned

Directions:

- ❖ Preheat oven to 400°F.
- ❖ Place the beef into a mixing bowl. Now, mix in the egg, salt, onion, garlic salt, Italian seasoning, oregano, red pepper flakes, hot pepper sauce, and Worcestershire sauce. Give it a good mix using your hand to evenly incorporate all the ingredients.
- ❖ Add parmesan cheese and bread crumbs.
- ❖ Mix until well combined and form ½ inch meatballs.
- ❖ Place the meatballs on to the baking sheets.

❖ Bake in the over for the next few minutes until the pink color of the uncooked meat is no longer seen
❖ Then cook for about 20-25 minutes.

Easy Marinated Shrimp
Serves 6-8
Calories 208, Protein 32g,
Total Fat 12g, Carbohydrates 1g, Fiber 0g

Ingredients:
❖ 3 minced garlic cloves
❖ 1/3 cup olive oil
❖ 1 tbsp. dry mustard
❖ 2 lbs. fresh shrimp, deveined, and peeled
❖ ¼ cup lemon juice
❖ ¼ cup fresh basil, chopped
❖ ½ tsp. salt

Directions:
❖ Take a large bowl and mix in the olive oil, dry mustard, lemon juice, and basil.
❖ Add the shrimp to the mixture and coat evenly.
❖ Cover the bowl with a cling film and refrigerate it for the next 2 to 4 hours.
❖ When ready to cook, preheat the oven to 350°F. Bake it for 6 to 8 minutes.
❖ Serve with salad.

Lobster Risotto with Asparagus

Serves 4
Calories 339, Protein 21g,
Total Fat 8g, Carbohydrates 43g, Fiber 1g

Ingredients:

- ❖ 4 frozen lobster tails
- ❖ 3 cups of vegetable broth (low sodium)
- ❖ 1 cup clam sauce
- ❖ 2 bay leaves
- ❖ 1 cup Arborio rice
- ❖ ½ cup white wine
- ❖ 1 medium-sized onion, finely chopped
- ❖ 1 shallot finely chopped
- ❖ 2 tbsp.butter
- ❖ 2 crushed garlic cloves
- ❖ 2 tbsp. of olive oil
- ❖ Salt & pepper to taste
- ❖ 1 cup chopped asparagus
- ❖ ½ cup fresh grated parmesan cheese
- ❖ Lemon (optional)

Directions:

- ❖ In a large pot over medium heat, heat 1 tbsp.olive oil and then add the shallot. Sauté for about 2 to 4 minutes until translucent.
- ❖ Add vegetable broth, clam sauce, bay leaves, and frozen uncooked lobster tails. Cover and cook over medium heat for 10 to 13 minutes. Remove lobster tails from the broth and let them cool. When they're

cool, dice into small pieces and set them aside. Set aside all remaining broth.

❖ In heated skillet, add 1 tbsp.olive oil and butter.

❖ Add the onion, garlic and sauté for about 3 to 5 minutes until the onion softens and starts changing its color.

❖ Add the Arborio rice and stir it for 1 minute.

❖ Gradually add half a cup of broth at a time and stir until the rice has absorbed almost all the broth.

❖ Add the asparagus and lobster with the wine and cook until the asparagus is tender. About 2 to 4 minutes.

❖ Stir in the parmesan cheese, salt, and pepper to taste.

❖ Squeeze lemon over top for an added zing, enjoy!

Vegan Macaroni and Cheese Bake
Serves 4
Calories 270, Protein 15g,
Total Fat 5g, Carbohydrates 50g, Fiber 8g

Ingredients:
 ❖ 1 cup of cashew nuts
 ❖ 1 cup of hot water
 ❖ 1 packet gluten-free pasta
 ❖ 1/3 cup nutritional yeast
 ❖ 1 tbsp. Dijon mustard
 ❖ 1 tsp. apple cider vinegar
 ❖ 2 crushed garlic cloves
 ❖ ½ medium onion, chopped finely
 ❖ 1 cup fresh kale chopped in a food processor

❖ ¼ tsp. cayenne pepper

Topping mix:
❖ For the topping, mix 1/3 cup of gluten-free breadcrumbs with ¼ cup vegan parmesan cheese, and 3 tbsp. of melted vegan butter.

Directions:
❖ Preheat oven to 350°F.
❖ Soak the cashews in hot water for 15 – 20 minutes.
❖ In a blender or food processor, mix the cashews and with hot water.
❖ Add the nutritional yeast, mustard, vinegar, garlic, onion, and cayenne pepper.
❖ Cook gluten-free pasta per package directions (directions will vary based on the type of gluten-free pasta selected).
❖ Drain the pasta and add in the cashew sauce and the kale.
❖ Place all ingredients in an 8x8 inch baking dish.
❖ Sprinkle topping mix over the baking dish and bake for about 20 minutes.

Vegetarian Crock Pot Chili
Serves 4
Calories 174, Protein 8g,
Total Fat 1g, Carbohydrates 33g, Fiber 9g

Ingredients:
- 1 can (14 oz.) black beans (organic in a BPA free can)
- 1 can (14 oz.) kidney beans (organic in a BPA free can)
- 1 can (28 oz.) tomatoes (organic in a BPA free can)
- ½ cup organic corn niblets
- 5 ½ oz. sundried tomato puree (see recipe below) or use store-bought tomato paste
- 2 tsp. chili powder
- 1 tsp. cumin
- 3 crushed garlic cloves
- 2 carrots, chopped in a food processor
- 1 onion, diced
- Dash of red pepper flakes
- 1 cup Gardein beefless ground
- 1 finely sliced green bell pepper
- 1 tsp. dried oregano

Directions:
- Add all the ingredients *except* the green peppers to the crockpot and cook on low heat for 6 hours.
- Top with green pepper and serve
- Optional side: jasmine rice, or gluten-free baked bread.

Sundried Tomato Puree Recipe
Ingredients:
- ❖ 1 (7 oz.) jar sun-dried tomatoes packed in oil, drained
- ❖ 5 cloves crushed garlic
- ❖ 2 to 4 tbsp.extra virgin olive oil
- ❖ 1 tsp. crushed oregano
- ❖ salt & freshly ground black pepper

Directions:
- ❖ In a food processor, add the tomatoes, garlic, seasonings, and oil and give it a good blend until a thick puree is formed. It can be refrigerated for up to 2 weeks.

Oven Roasted Vegetarian Stuffed Red Bell Peppers
Serves 4
Calories 254, Protein 12g,
Total Fat 4g, Carbohydrates 44g, Fiber 8g

Ingredients:
- ❖ 4 red bell peppers, seeded and top sliced off
- ❖ 2 cups cooked quinoa (cooked per package instructions)
- ❖ 1 can (14 ounces) of black beans, thoroughly rinsed and drained
- ❖ ½ sweet onion, diced
- ❖ 1 tomato, diced
- ❖ 1 tsp. chili powder

- ❖ ½ tsp. cumin
- ❖ 1 garlic clove (minced)
- ❖ 1 tsp. salt
- ❖ 1 pinch ground black pepper
- ❖ ¼ cup shredded Mexican cheese blend

Directions:
- ❖ Preheat oven to 375°F.
- ❖ Top the baking sheet with parchment paper.
- ❖ Place the peppers cut-side down on the baking sheet.
- ❖ Roast the peppers for 3 to 4 minutes until the skin starts to brown. Remove from oven
- ❖ In a nonstick skillet, heat the oil over medium heat.
- ❖ Add the onions, garlic, chili powder, cumin, salt, and pepper to the skillet and cook for the next 2 to 3 minutes.
- ❖ Stir in the black beans and tomato and cook for another 5 to 7 minutes.
- ❖ Add in the cooked quinoa and stir until it's thoroughly heated.
- ❖ Spoon the mixture into the bell pepper halves made out like cups.
- ❖ Top it with shredded cheese.
- ❖ Place in the oven and bake for 25 to 30 minutes. Serve immediately.

French Canadian Tourtiere

Serves 5 - 6
Calories 405, Protein 15g,
Total Fat 27 g, Carbohydrates 26g, Fiber 2g

Ingredients:
- ❖ 1 lb. of lean ground pork.
- ❖ 1 lb. of lean ground beef
- ❖ 1 onion, diced
- ❖ 2 garlic cloves
- ❖ ½ tsp. ground thyme
- ❖ ¼ tsp. ground sage
- ❖ 1/8 tsp. ground cloves
- ❖ Salt & pepper to taste
- ❖ 2 (9-inch) gluten-free pie crusts

Directions:
- ❖ Preheat the oven to 425°F.
- ❖ Heat a skillet and add the pork, beef, onion, garlic thyme, sage, pepper, and cloves. Simmer until the mixture boils.
- ❖ Reduce the heat and cook it for another 5 to 6 minutes.
- ❖ Drain the mixture and spoon into the pie crust.
- ❖ Top the pie with the second pie crust. Cut slits into the top pie crust in order to allow steam to escape. Pinch the edge of the pie crust to seal the pie.
- ❖ Cover the edge with an aluminum foil so that it doesn't burn.
- ❖ Bake for 20 minutes.

❖ Reduce the heat to 375°F, remove the foil from the edge and bake for an additional 20 to 25 minutes.

Chapter 8
Healthy Snacks

Snacking is a healthy way to fit in extra nutrients to your diet and prevent yourself from overeating at mealtimes.

Being healthy doesn't always mean just being skinny, it has a more in-depth meaning to it. Some people may avoid eating snacks because they think it might increase their weight. But the lesser-known fact is that opting for a healthy snack with balanced nutrients can actually contribute to weight loss. According to a study, 97% of Americans snack and get about 24% of their calorie intake from snacking.

Consuming healthy snacks in between your meals may lead to many direct and indirect health benefits, including:

- ❖ Increased level of nutrient intake
- ❖ Appetite Control
- ❖ Better concentration of the mind
- ❖ Increased level of energy

Healthy snacking improves your overall health, curbs cravings because you do not get hungry at odd times. Moreover, consuming healthy snacks helps fight against weight gain, regulates mood, boosts brainpower and gives you the energy that you need to keep going all day long. It maintains consistent energy sourcing throughout the day so that you feel refreshed and don't get worn out by the end of the day.

Pro-tip: prepare your snacks ahead of time and store them for later in order to satisfy hunger pangs occurring at odd times of the day. Moreover, preparing ahead of time also allows you to stick to your healthy diet plan. But if you don't have a diet plan, then you can make one instantly when required. Therefore, it is imperative to remember that the snacks should be simple, not so complex in terms of preparation, and ready to be cooked without consuming more of your time.

For healthy snacks, you can opt from a wide variety of choices ranging from various types of refreshing sports drinks, salad dressing, sandwiches or other wholefood snacks with sweet and savory combinations.

Healthy Breakfast Smoothie

Serves 1
Calories 225, Protein 21.3, Total Fat 6.3g, Carbohydrates 22.1g, Fiber 2.3g

Ingredients:
- ❖ 1 medium-sized banana (fresh or frozen)
- ❖ ½ cup fresh fruit (strawberries, mangoes or blueberries)
- ❖ ¼ cup of plain Greek yogurt
- ❖ 1 tbsp. almond butter
- ❖ ½ cup baby spinach
- ❖ ½ cup almond milk
- ❖ 2-3 mint leaves (to garnish)

Directions:
- ❖ Add in all the ingredients in a blender and blend until smooth.
- ❖ Garnish with mint leaves and serve.

Red Wine Berry Spritzer

Serves 1
Calories 137, Protein 0.6g, Total Fat 0.2g, Carbohydrates 13.1g, Fiber 1.6g

Ingredients:
- ❖ 1 part red wine
- ❖ 2 parts Sparkling Water
- ❖ Ice
- ❖ Frozen berries of your choice (blueberries or raspberries)

Directions:
- ❖ Add frozen berries to the bottom of a glass and smash in the glass.
- ❖ Add ice and pour wine and sparkling water.
- ❖ Stir, sip and enjoy.

Detox Water – Fruit Infused Water

Serves 4
Calories 27, Protein 0.6g, Total Fat 0g, Carbohydrates 6.8g, Fiber 1.5g

Ingredients:
- ❖ 1 orange, thinly sliced
- ❖ 5 to 7 strawberries, sliced thinly
- ❖ A handful of fresh mint leaves (washed and rinsed)
- ❖ 1 jug of water

Directions:
- ❖ Place the sliced fruits and mint leaves in a jug.
- ❖ Pour water and refrigerate for at least 1-2 hours. The more it sits, the more flavorful the water becomes.
- ❖ Drink it throughout the day.
- ❖ Change fruits after every 12 hours, or just pop them into the blender for a tropical smoothie.

ApfelSchorle
Serves 4
Calories 246, Protein 0.4g, Total Fat 22.7g,
Carbohydrates 12.6g, Fiber 0.3g

Ingredients:
- ❖ 4 cups fresh apple juice (from the juicer)
- ❖ 4 cups of bottle-carbonated mineral water

Directions:
- ❖ Mix equal parts of apple juice and carbonated water in a tall glass.
- ❖ Garnish with a slice of lemon.

Pumpkin Smoothie
Serves 2
Calories 211, Protein 8.8g, Total Fat 3.7g, Carbohydrates 35.9g, Fiber 3.3g

Ingredients:
- ❖ 1 cup milk
- ❖ ½ cup pumpkin puree
- ❖ ½ cup yogurt
- ❖ 1 tbsp. maple syrup
- ❖ ¼ tsp. pumpkin pie spice
- ❖ Splash vanilla
- ❖ 1 frozen banana

Directions:
- ❖ Combine all the ingredients into a blender at once.
- ❖ Give it a good blend until the mixture reaches the uniform consistency.

Portobello Mushroom Frics
Serves 2
Calories 217, Protein 10.8g, Total Fat 5.1g,
Carbohydrates 32.2g, Fiber 2.3g

Ingredients:
- ❖ 2 medium Portobello mushrooms gills removed, sliced ¼ inch thick
- ❖ 2 medium eggs at room temperature, slightly beaten
- ❖ ¾ cup breadcrumbs (gluten-free)
- ❖ ¾ cup grated parmesan cheese
- ❖ 1 tsp. Montreal steak spice
- ❖ ½ tsp. thyme
- ❖ Salt
- ❖ ½ cup extra virgin olive oil

Directions:
- ❖ Cut mushrooms into ¼ inch strips.
- ❖ In one bowl, beat the eggs. In a separate bowl mix breadcrumbs, parmesan cheese, steak spice, salt, and pepper. Dip the mushroom strips into the egg mixture, then into the breadcrumb mixture.
- ❖ Heat the oil and, once heated, add the mushrooms turning every 3 minutes. Cook until they are crispy (about 8-12 minutes).

Smoky Kale Chips

Serves 2
Calories 175, Protein 6.9g, Total Fat 7.1g, Carbohydrates 24.3g, Fiber 3.8g

Ingredients:
- ❖ 1 lb. Kale
- ❖ 1 tbsp. extra virgin olive oil
- ❖ 1 tsp. smoked paprika
- ❖ ¼ tsp. salt

Directions:
- ❖ Preheat oven to 350°F.
- ❖ Wash and rinse the kale thoroughly and dry it onto a paper towel.
- ❖ Remove the stems from the leaves and tear the leaves into 3-4 inch pieces.
- ❖ Toss the kale with extra virgin olive oil, paprika powder, and salt. Make sure all the leaves are coated evenly with the oil and seasoning.
- ❖ Spread the coated leaves onto a baking sheet and place them in the oven.
- ❖ Bake at 350°F until the edges turn brown and crispy for about 12-15 minutes.

Tomato, Mozzarella and Basil Bruschetta

Makes 8-10
Calories 124, Protein 6g, Total Fat 6g, Carbohydrates 12g, Fiber 1g

Ingredients:
- ❖ 4 cups cherry tomatoes
- ❖ ½ avocado
- ❖ ½ onion
- ❖ 1 cup fresh basil
- ❖ 4 tbsp. extra virgin olive oil
- ❖ 6 garlic cloves, peeled
- ❖ Salt
- ❖ Pepper
- ❖ 2 large gluten-free baguettes, 1-inch thick
- ❖ 1 ½ lb. mozzarella cheese

Directions:
- ❖ Preheat oven to 375°F.
- ❖ Add tomatoes, garlic, onion, basil, avocado, and olive oil into a food processor and pulse until the paste becomes a little chunky.
- ❖ Season it with salt and pepper.
- ❖ Toast your baguette slices on a baking sheet for 3 to 4 minutes until reached desired crisp.
- ❖ Lay a slice of mozzarella cheese on top of each slice and put it back into the oven for the next 5 to 6 minutes or until the cheese has melted.
- ❖ Remove the baguettes from the oven and spread the chunky tomato paste evenly on top of that.

❖ Serve the bruschetta on a plate and garnish it with basil leaves.

Summer Avocado Shrimp Crostini

Serves 6-8

Calories 256, Protein 25g, Total Fat 12.5g, Carbohydrates 10g, Fiber 0g

Ingredients:

❖ 1 lb. cooked shrimp, deveined, peeled and diced
❖ 1 avocado mashed and chunky
❖ juice and zest of 1 lime
❖ ¼ cup finely diced red onion
❖ ¼ cup chopped cilantro
❖ ¼ cup chopped chives
❖ ¼ tsp. cumin
❖ Pinch of crushed chili pepper
❖ Salt to taste

Directions:

❖ In a small bowl mix lime juice and zest, avocado, red onion, cilantro, chives, cumin, chili pepper, and salt.
❖ Toss shrimp in this mixture and give them a good coat of flavors.
❖ Gently press each shrimp in breadcrumbs in a separate bowl and coat it evenly from both sides.
❖ Spread mixture onto individual crostini. Garnish with chives.

Mixed Veggies with Avocado-Cilantro Dip

Serves 4
Calories 240, Protein 7g, Total Fat 18g, Carbohydrates 18g, Fiber 8g

Ingredients:
- ❖ 1 head cauliflower, sliced into cross-sections (stem removed)
- ❖ 1 English cucumber, sliced into spears
- ❖ 2 celery stalks, sliced in sticks
- ❖ ½ cup cream cheese
- ❖ ½ cup chopped cilantro
- ❖ 10 grape tomatoes
- ❖ 1 tbsp. lime juice
- ❖ 1 avocado, peeled
- ❖ 1/8 tsp. cayenne (optional)
- ❖ Salt and Pepper

Directions:
- ❖ Place the cut vegetables on a serving platter.
- ❖ In a food processor, add the cream cheese, cilantro, grape tomatoes, lime juice, avocado, and cayenne.
- ❖ Blend until the paste becomes smooth and creamy.
- ❖ Season with salt and pepper.
- ❖ Transfer to a dip bowl and serve with cauliflower, cucumber, and celery.

Fro-Yo Berry Bites

Serves 6-8
Calories 73, Protein 3.7g, Total Fat 2.3g, Carbohydrates 13g, Fiber 1.3g

Ingredients:

- ❖ 4 cups of plain Greek Yogurt
- ❖ 4 tablespoons of honey
- ❖ ¼ cup raisins
- ❖ ¼ cup chopped almonds
- ❖ 1 tsp. vanilla extract
- ❖ 1 orange, zest grated
- ❖ ¼ cup of orange juice
- ❖ Berries of your choice (Blueberries, Raspberries, or strawberries)

Directions:

- ❖ Line a sieve with cheesecloth and place it in a bowl.
- ❖ Pour in your yogurt and let it drain all the moisture for better consistency.
- ❖ Refrigerate the yogurt for the next 3 to 4 hours.
- ❖ Pour the yogurt into a separate bowl and mix in the orange juice and honey. Mix until all the ingredients are well combined. Add orange juice gradually to reach the desired consistency.
- ❖ Toss in the almonds, raisins, berries, and orange zest.
- ❖ Pour the liquid yogurt into the ice-cube tray and let it sit in the freezer overnight.
- ❖ Enjoy your Fro-Yo Berry Bites chilled.

Stuffed Honey & Almond Butter Apple

Serves 2
Calories 224, Protein 7g, Total Fat 12.1g, Carbohydrates 39.4g, Fiber 5.5g

Ingredients:
- ❖ 1 apple, washed and cored
- ❖ 2 tbsp. almond butter
- ❖ 2 tbsp. granola
- ❖ ½ tsp. coconut oil
- ❖ honey

Directions:
- ❖ Preheat the oven to 325°F
- ❖ Wash and hollow out the apple.
- ❖ Mix the almond butter and granola.
- ❖ Top the apple with the coconut oil and bake for 20 minutes.
- ❖ Remove from the oven and drizzle with honey.
- ❖ Place on a serving tray and serve immediately.

Cashew Cherry Energy Bites

Serves 3
Calories 345, Protein 3.9g, Total Fat 7.3g, Carbohydrates 53.4g, Fiber 14.4g

Ingredients:
- ❖ ½ cup dried cherries
- ❖ 1/3 cup raw cashews
- ❖ ¼ tsp. vanilla
- ❖ 1 tsp. flax seed

❖ 2 dates

Directions:
- ❖ Toss the cashews into a food processor to break them into smaller pieces.
- ❖ Add flaxseed to the food processor and pulse until they are broken into small pieces as well.
- ❖ Add the remaining ingredients in the food processor and pulse until they begin to stick together.
- ❖ With a slightly damp palm, take 2 tbsp. of the mixture and roll it between your both palms, making a ball.
- ❖ Continue this process until all of the mixtures have been rolled.
- ❖ The energy bites are ready to be served.

Dark Chocolate Detox Medley

Makes 24
Calories 55, Protein 0.8g, Total Fat 2.8g, Carbohydrates 6.7g, Fiber 0.5g

Ingredients:
- ❖ 8 oz. of dark chocolate
- ❖ 1 cup assorted dried fruits, chopped nuts and seeds (ie: slivered almonds, candied ginger, chia, dried cranberries, pumpkin seeds)

Directions:
- ❖ Cut out a sheet of parchment paper and place it into a tray.

- ❖ Chop the dark chocolate into smaller chunks or grate it.
- ❖ Heat the chocolate in a double boiler until the chocolate is completely melted.
- ❖ Use a spoon to make small rounds of chocolate onto the parchment paper layout.
- ❖ Place in your choice of assortment nuts, fruit, and seeds on the chocolate circle while the chocolate is still hot.
- ❖ Let the chocolate set at room temperature or you can put the bites in the refrigerator. Enjoy!

Fresh Mango and Berry Salad

Serves 4 - 6
Calories 128, Protein 4.2g, Total Fat 1.4g, Carbohydrates 74.4g, Fiber 15.2g

Ingredients:
- ❖ 1 mango, peeled and cubed
- ❖ 1 cup sliced strawberries
- ❖ 1 cup raspberries or blueberries
- ❖ 2 kiwis, peeled and cubed
- ❖ 1 banana sliced
- ❖ 2 seedless navel oranges
- ❖ 3 tbsp. honey (optional)

Directions:
- ❖ Mix all ingredients together.
- ❖ Refrigerate it for at least one hour before serving.
- ❖ Top with honey if desired. Serve chilled.

Chapter 9
Sides

Side dishes are awesome. People do not appreciate how the flavors of a side dish can enhance your main course. The right side dish needs extra prep work for a healthy reward. However, choosing the right side dish makes all the difference to your main course.

Adding a side of fruits or vegetables is a great way to incorporate healthy fruits and vegetables into your meal. These nutrients are essential for our diet. You can also add a salad to your main course for the perfect balance. The possibilities are endless, and the benefits are uncountable.

Roasted Root Vegetables
Serves 4
170 Calories, 12.5g Carbs(12.5g net carbs), 4.5g Fat, 27g
Protein, *Fiber 5.3g*

Ingredients:
* ❖ 10 beets (optional: carrots, red onion, and potatoes)
* ❖ 4 tbsp. of extra virgin olive oil
* ❖ 2 tsp. fresh thyme leaves, finely chopped
* ❖ 2 tsp. salt
* ❖ 2 tbsp. apple cider vinegar

Directions:
* ❖ Preheat the oven to 400ºF.
* ❖ Cut off the tops and roots of the beets and peel them using a vegetable peeler.
* ❖ Cut the beets (and other vegetables) into bite-size chunks.
* ❖ In a separate bowl, mix together olive oil, thyme, vinegar, and salt.
* ❖ Toss in the beet chunks and stir until each piece is well coated.
* ❖ Place the cut beets on a baking sheet and roast them for 35 to 40 minutes until tender.
* ❖ Turn the beets halfway through cooking time.
* ❖ Remove the beets from the oven and transfer them to a bowl.

* ❖ Serve hot.

Roasted Asparagus

Serves 4

Calories 95, Protein 3g, Total Fat 8g, Carbohydrates 4g, Fiber 1g

Ingredients:
- ❖ 1 lb. fresh asparagus, trimmed
- ❖ 1 cup grape tomatoes, halved (optional)
- ❖ 1 tbsp. of pine nuts (optional)
- ❖ 1 ½ tbsp. olive oil
- ❖ 1 crushed garlic clove
- ❖ Kosher salt
- ❖ Pepper
- ❖ 1 tbsp. of lime juice
- ❖ grated parmesan cheese
- ❖ ½ tsp. lemon zest

Directions:
- ❖ Preheat the oven to 400°F.
- ❖ In a separate bowl mix in olive oil, garlic, salt, and pepper. Give it a good mix.
- ❖ Now toss in your pine nuts, asparagus, and tomatoes to coat them evenly.
- ❖ Bake it for the next 15 minutes until the asparagus is tender.
- ❖ Squeeze a lemon over the top of your veggies and nuts.
- ❖ Top it all with some grated cheese and lemon zest to enhance the flavor.

Pan-Roasted Brussel Sprouts with Bacon

Serves 4
Calories 210, Protein 11.2g, Total Fat 14.1g,
Carbohydrates 12.4g, Fiber 4.7g

Ingredients:
- ❖ 4 bacon strips (thick cut)
- ❖ 2 tbsp. of unsalted butter
- ❖ 1 lb. Brussel sprouts halved
- ❖ 1 medium onion, chopped
- ❖ Salt and pepper to taste

Directions:
- ❖ Cook Bacon strips on high heat in a nonstick pan or iron skillet until crispy.
- ❖ Place them onto a paper towel until the excess oil is absorbed.
- ❖ Chop the bacon strips.
- ❖ In the same pan, add butter on medium-high heat. Once melted, add chopped onions and Brussel sprouts, and cook until golden brown.
- ❖ Season the sprouts with some salt and pepper.
- ❖ Toss the bacon back into the pan and serve hot.

Creamy Mashed Cauliflower

Serves 4
Calories 107, Protein 5g, Total Fat 7g, Carbohydrates 10g, Fiber 4g

Ingredients:

- ❖ 1 head cauliflower cut into bite-sized florets (stems removed)
- ❖ 4 garlic cloves
- ❖ 4 tsp. of olive oil
- ❖ 1 tbsp. of butter (or vegan butter)
- ❖ 1 tbsp. nutritional yeast
- ❖ a pinch of salt
- ❖ Chives to garnish

Directions:

- ❖ Place the garlic and cauliflower in a steamer over 1-inch of boiling water. Cover and steam until tender —approximately 8 minutes.
- ❖ Drain cauliflower.

Using an immersion blender, add olive oil, butter, nutritional yeast, and salt and blend until desired texture is reached.

Roasted Broccoli with Garlic

Serves 4
Calories 111, Protein 5g, Total Fat 8g, Carbohydrates 10g, Fiber 5g

Ingredients:
- ❖ 1 bunch of broccoli (cut into florets)
- ❖ 2 tbsp. of extra virgin olive oil
- ❖ juice of half a lemon
- ❖ 3 chopped garlic cloves
- ❖ sea salt

Directions:
- ❖ Preheat oven to 450°F.
- ❖ In a separate bowl, mix olive oil, salt, garlic, and lemon.
- ❖ Toss in the broccoli florets and give them a good shake so that each piece gets evenly coated.
- ❖ Spread them on the baking sheet and place them in the oven for 15-20 minutes or until the broccoli gets that outer thin crisp and inner tender part. Watch closely so that it doesn't burn.
- ❖ Serve warm.

Baked Salt & Paprika Fries

Serves 4
Calories 280, Protein 6g, Total Fat 7g, Carbohydrates 50g, Fiber 3.6g

Ingredients:
- ❖ 3 to 4 large organic potatoes
- ❖ 3 tbsp. olive oil
- ❖ ¼ tsp. paprika (optional)
- ❖ Salt

Directions:
- ❖ Preheat the oven to 450ºF.
- ❖ Cut the potatoes into uniform julienne pieces.
- ❖ In a large bowl, mix the olive oil, salt, and paprika. Give it a good mix until all spices are combined.
- ❖ Toss in your cut potatoes and shake the bowl to coat every piece evenly.
- ❖ Spread the coated fries on a baking sheet and bake until they become golden and crispy. About 35 minutes. Turn the fries about halfway through baking.
- ❖ Serve them as it is or with a guacamole dip.

Zucchini and Mushroom Stir-fry

Serves 4-6
Calories 286, Protein 5g, Total Fat 16.5g, Carbohydrates 28g, Fiber 1g

Ingredients:

- 3 zucchini (diced into ½ inch pieces)
- 1 onion, diced
- 16 ounces sliced mushrooms (stems removed)
- 1 cup broccoli (optional)
- 1 tsp. Worcestershire sauce
- ¼ cup white wine
- 2 cloves garlic, crushed
- 3 tbsp. unsalted butter
- Salt
- Ground black pepper

Directions:

- ❖ Melt the butter in a large skillet over medium-high heat.
- ❖ Add the diced onion and sauté until it begins to soften about 2 minutes.
- ❖ Stir in garlic and thyme and sauté for another minute.
- ❖ Add mushrooms and cook for 5 minutes or until they begin to soften. There should be water from the mushrooms in the skillet.
- ❖ Add in the zucchini and sauté for another 2 minutes.
- ❖ Add white wine and stir it for one more minute.
- ❖ Serve immediately.

Note: For a thicker sauce, mix 1 tbsp. corn starch with 2 ounces of water. Remove vegetables from liquid. Bring the liquid to a boil and slowly incorporate the cornstarch mixture. If the sauce becomes too thick, add a little more white wine and water.

Coriander-Maple Glazed Carrots

Serves 4
Calories 143, Protein 2.1g, Total Fat 7g, Carbohydrates 19.6g, Fiber 4.1g

Ingredients:
- ❖ 1 ½ rainbow carrots, halved crosswise
- ❖ 2 tbsp. olive oil
- ❖ 2 tsp. whole coriander seeds, crushed
- ❖ Kosher salt
- ❖ Ground black pepper
- ❖ ¾ tbsp. pure maple syrup
- ❖ 1 tsp. lemon zest
- ❖ 1 tbsp. lemon juice

Directions:
- ❖ Heat oven to 425°F.
- ❖ Toss the carrots, oil and coriander seeds in a separate bowl.
- ❖ sprinkle over some salt and pepper.
- ❖ Divide the carrots into two baking sheets and bake in the bottom and middle positions.
- ❖ Stir in between baking until golden brown and tender.
- ❖ Toss with maple syrup and lime zest and juice.

Apple, Beet and Fennel Salad Recipe

Serves 4
Calories 224, Protein 2.2g, Total Fat 13.1g, Carbohydrates 28.5g, Fiber 6.9g

Ingredients:

- ❖ 3 small-sized beets
- ❖ ½ small fennel bulb, halved lengthwise
- ❖ ½ medium-sized apple
- ❖ 3 cups packed arugula
- ❖ 2-3 tbsp. flat-leaf parsley
- ❖ 4-5 fresh mint leaves fresh mint leaves
- ❖ 3 tbsp. of olive oil
- ❖ 1 tbsp. of apple cider vinegar
- ❖ ¾ tsp. orange zest
- ❖ ¾ tbsp. fresh orange juice
- ❖ ¼ tsp. kosher salt
- ❖ ½ tsp. honey
- ❖ a pinch of black pepper (powder)

Directions:

- ❖ Place beets in a medium saucepan with chilled water.
- ❖ Place the saucepan over high heat and bring the water to a boil.
- ❖ Reduce the heat to medium and let it simmer until the beets are fork-tender.
- ❖ Once done, drain the water and let them sit out to cool.
- ❖ Now Peel the beets and cut into wedges.

❖ Cut the fennel bulb and apples into very thin slices. Place in a large bowl with beet wedges, arugula, parsley, and mint.
❖ In a large bowl, whisk together vinegar, oil, zest, juice, honey, salt, and black pepper.
❖ Drizzle the vinaigrette over the beet mixture toss to coat evenly.
❖ Serve immediately.

Spice-Roasted Butternut Squash with Cider Vinegar

Serves 4
Calories 135, Protein 1g, Total Fat10g, Carbohydrates 11g, Fiber 2g

Ingredients:

❖ 1 tsp. light brown sugar
❖ ½ ground coriander
❖ ¼ tsp. freshly grated nutmeg
❖ 1 small butternut squash (seeded, peeled and sliced into half-inch-thick wedges)
❖ 2 tsp. of fresh thyme
❖ 3-4 tbsp. of extra virgin olive oil.
❖ ½ cup apple cider
❖ ½ tbsp. red wine vinegar
❖ ½ tbsp. whole grain mustard
❖ 2 tbsp. of parsley leaves (chopped)
❖ Kosher salt
❖ Pinch of grounded black pepper

Directions:

- ❖ Preheat the oven to 425°F.
- ❖ In a separate bowl mix in coriander, sugar, nutmeg, and a pinch of salt and pepper.
- ❖ Divide squash and thyme between 2 large baking sheets.
- ❖ Toss vegetables on each sheet with oil, and half of the spice mixture. Arrange the vegetables in a single layer and roast until golden brown and tender. Transfer to a platter.
- ❖ Heat the cider on high heat in a saucepan.
- ❖ Reduce the heat and simmer until liquid has reduced to half.
- ❖ In a separate bowl, whisk together your vinegar, cider, mustard, oil and salt and pepper.
- ❖ Stir in the parsley and drizzle over the squash.

Garlic Butter Roasted Butternut Squash

Serves 4
Calories 166, Protein 0.3g, Total Fat 12.8g, Carbohydrates 1.1g, Fiber 0.1g

Ingredients:

- 1 large butternut squash (peeled, seeded)
- 2 tbsp. of salted butter on room temperature
- 2 tbsp. of extra virgin olive oil
- 4 garlic cloves finely chopped
- a pinch of salt
- ½ tsp. Of Cajun Seasoning.
- ½ tbsp. of ground black pepper
- Fresh Parsley (chopped)

Directions:

- Prepare the oven and preheat it to 420°F.
- Cut the butternut squash into two halves and deseed it.
- Brush it with olive oil and sprinkle some salt and pepper.
- Place the butternut squash cut side down on the baking sheet and roast until softened.
- In a separate bowl mix in olive oil, melted butter, Cajun seasoning, garlic, and ground black pepper. Set this aside.
- Take out the squash from the oven, let sit for 2 minutes and then transfer it to the cutting board.
- With a sharp knife, cut slits in the squash.
- Brush it with the garlic butter Cajun sauce and transfer it to the baking sheet. Make sure to coat well and between the slices.
- Roast it in the oven for the next 25-30 minutes.
- Serve the squash with chopped parsley and sprinkle kosher salt.

Cauliflower Breadsticks

Ingredients:
- ❖ 1 head of cauliflower (riced)
- ❖ 1 tsp. oregano
- ❖ 2 garlic cloves, crushed
- ❖ 2 large eggs
- ❖ ¼ cup grated parmesan
- ❖ ½ cup + 1 cup shredded cheese for topping (I like cheddar but you can also use mozzarella or pizza mix cheese)

Directions:
- ❖ Preheat the oven to 425 F.
- ❖ Line a baking sheet with a parchment paper.
- ❖ Break the cauliflower into florets, remove and discard the stem.
- ❖ Steam in ½ inch of boiling water (covered) until soft. About 7 minutes
- ❖ Place the florets in the food processor and pulse it until the texture of the cauliflower looks similar to rice. (Squeeze the riced, raw cauliflower in cheesecloth or a clean towel to help remove moisture.)
- ❖ In a separate bowl, mix the cauliflower, parmesan cheese, ½ cup shredded or grated cheese, eggs, garlic, oregano, and salt until combined and holds together.
- ❖ Place the mixture and pour it into the lined baking sheet. Spread it out evenly in a rectangular 9x7 inch baking sheet and ¼ inch thick.
- ❖ Bake it in the oven for the next 10-12 minutes.

❖ Take it out from the oven and top it with the shredded cheese. Now, put it back in the oven and continue baking until the cheese is melted and golden on the top.
❖ Let it cool for about 10 minutes and then cut it into breadsticks.
❖ Garnish the dish with fresh herbs and parmesan cheese. Serve hot and enjoy!

Stir Fried Green Beans

Serves 4
Calories 123, Protein 4.3g, Total Fat 6.1g, Carbohydrates 16.7g, Fiber 7.9g

Ingredients:
❖ 1 small chopped onion
❖ 2 lbs. green beans, trimmed
❖ 2 tbsp. butter
❖ 2 tbsp. melted butter
❖ Salt

Directions:
❖ Fill a pan with water about 2 inches high and bring it to simmer.
❖ Add the beans.
❖ Cook covered for 3 minutes. Make sure the beans retain their bright green color.
❖ Drain the beans.
❖ Saute the onions in a saucepan with melted butter and salt until the onions are soft.

❖ Add the steamed green beans and saute for 2 more minutes.
❖ Serve warm.

Roasted Carrots and Parsnips

Serves 4

Calories 157, Protein 1.6g, Total Fat 10.6g, Carbohydrates 16g, Fiber 4g

Ingredients:
❖ 5 carrots
❖ 5 parsnips
❖ 1 red onion chopped
❖ 3 tbsp. of extra virgin olive oil
❖ 1 tsp. fresh thyme
❖ 1 ¼ tsp. Of regular salt
❖ Dash of ground pepper
❖ 2 tbsp. fresh rosemary

Directions:
❖ Prepare your oven for half an hour, preheat it to 400ºF.
❖ Cut the carrots, parsnips, and onion diagonally into 2-inch pieces.
❖ Toss them in a bowl with olive oil, thyme, salt, and pepper and coat it evenly.
❖ Transfer it to the baking sheet and roast it in the oven for the next 20 minutes, until brown and tender.
❖ Sprinkles fresh rosemary on the top of the veggies to serve.

Farinata (Italian Chickpea Pancake)

Serves 4
Calories 105.6, Protein 3.5g, Total Fat 6.2g, Carbohydrates 8.8g, Fiber 1.7g

Ingredients:
- ❖ 1 ¾ cups of finely ground chickpea flour
- ❖ 1 tsp. kosher salt
- ❖ 3 cups of water
- ❖ ¼ cup of extra virgin olive oil
- ❖ Freshly ground pepper
- ❖ Rosemary leaves, for sprinkling

Directions:
- ❖ In a large bowl, mix the chickpea flour and salt together.
- ❖ Gradually add water, little at a time constantly whisking until it forms a smooth, thin batter.
- ❖ Cover the batter with a damp cloth or cling film and let stand for 4-8 hours.
- ❖ Preheat the oven to 500ºF and place the oven rack in the second position from the top.
- ❖ Pour olive oil in a large nonstick skillet and spread evenly. Using a spoon, scrape any foam and discard.
- ❖ Stir the batter to mix well and pour into the skillet.
- ❖ Season it with some salt and pepper.
- ❖ Sprinkle over the chopped rosemary leaves.
- ❖ Turn on the broiler and cook until the farinata is set and is browned all over about 11 minutes.

❖ Let the farinata cool until set and eat warm or at room temperature.

Chapter 10
Healthy Desserts

When it comes to eating healthy, most people even despise the idea of consuming sweets. The rest wonders where they can fit in this sweet chunk of heaven in their healthy meal without feeling the guilt. It can be really challenging to stop one's self from raising the hand when it comes to the time for sweet. For sure, sweet is the part of a whole meal that completes the dinner with a happy ending.

Also, people with a sweet tooth can relate to the fact that you should not wait for any specific reason to eat sweet, you just do it. Well, let me tell you what, sweet can be the part of your daily meals, but the key to be healthy while consuming them is the proportion. A balanced amount of calorie consumption is all that it takes to convert craving into the essential source of energy.

If you control the quantity of sweetness in your sweet, you can satisfy your sweet tooth or salty cravings every day. To consume a special treat for more than a few hundred calories, make sure that you earn it by being a little extra active physically. Eat it as you have earned it.

To be able to incorporate sweets and treats in your diet, consider some of the ways suggested by experts:

- **Stock Up Healthy Choices** Every calorie counts, make sure the count is worth it. Don't just count the calories but keep the account of maintaining a balanced meal. Choose treats and desserts that have a total of 100-200 calories and contain nutritional benefits.

- **Go Natural for Dessert** There's nothing wrong in occasionally popping a spoonful of baked sweets such as cakes or Brule once or twice a week. But in order to be able to consume the sweets more frequently and not disrupting the healthy diet cycle, substitute your sweet base with natural products such as fruits and dry fruits. These desserts are so easy to overeat, and the small portion is not nearly as satisfying.

- **Limit the Variety of Sweets** Having a wide variety of choices may be the freedom of eating. However, when it comes to controlling calories, less is more. The wider the range of available foods and products, the more urge you have to eat. Therefore, it is best to keep the variety as minimal as possible.

• **Modify Your Recipes** Cooking is all about experimenting with the new tastes, ingredients, and flavors. Your kitchen is your laboratory where you can create wonders through new inventions. Always try finding a better, healthier substitute for your food. For example, instead of sugary or glucose-y sprinkles, top your cakes with dry fruits. Or, replace half the fats by substituting applesauce or canola oil in the baking of your favorite cake or cookie recipe and such.

Gluten-free Fruit Scones
Makes 8 scones
Calories 302, Protein 4g, Total Fat 13g, Carbohydrates 42g, Fiber 1g

Ingredients:
- ❖ 1 ¾ cup Gluten-free All-Purpose Flour
- ❖ ¼ cup coconut sugar
- ❖ 2 tsp. gluten-free baking powder
- ❖ ½ tsp. xantham gum
- ❖ A pinch of salt
- ❖ ¼ tsp. nutmeg
- ❖ ½ cup cold butter
- ❖ ¾ cup of diced fresh fruit
- ❖ 3 eggs at room temperature
- ❖ 1/3 cup of almond milk
- ❖ 1 tsp. pure vanilla bean extract

Directions:
- ❖ Preheat the oven to 400°F.
- ❖ Grease the divided scone pan (or mold).
- ❖ Whisk together all the dry ingredients such as flour, baking powder, salt, nutmeg, sugar, and xantham gum in a separate bowl. Now add the cold butter to the dry ingredients and mix it until the mixture is crumbly.
- ❖ Toss in the dried fruits.
- ❖ Now whisk all your dry ingredients in a separate bowl, including milk, eggs, and vanilla extract until the mixture becomes frothy.
- ❖ Now add this mixture to the dry ingredients until well blended and forms a dough.
- ❖ The dough should be stiff and should stick together or don't fall apart.
- ❖ Drop the dough by 1/3 cupful into the scone pan. Let the scones rest for the next 10 to 15 minutes until they rise a little bit in size.
- ❖ Drizzle the scones with some honey strands to add that spark of extra sweetness.
- ❖ Now, bake the scones for 15-20 minutes until golden brown.
- ❖ Now turn off the heat and let your scones sit in the oven for the next 5 minutes.
- ❖ After removing them from the oven, let them sit out for a while before you serve them on to the plates.
- ❖ Enjoy with butter and jam.

Gluten-free Cheddar Scone

Makes 8 scones

Calories 283, Protein 6g, Total Fat 15g, Carbohydrates 33g, Fiber 4g

Ingredients:
- ❖ 2 ½ cups Multipurpose flour (gluten-free)
- ❖ A pinch of. salt
- ❖ 1 tsp. Xanthan Gum
- ❖ 1 tsp. sugar
- ❖ 2 tsp. gluten-free baking powder
- ❖ 2/3 cup of almond or coconut milk
- ❖ 2 eggs
- ❖ 1/3 cup of vegan butter or shortening.
- ❖ 1 cup vegan cheddar shreds
- ❖ ¼ cup chopped chives

Directions:
- ❖ Preheat the oven to 350°F.
- ❖ Blend all the gluten-free all-purpose flour, sugar, salt, baking powder, and Xanthan Gum in a bowl.
- ❖ Once all the dry ingredients are blended, add in the vegan butter, cheddar shreds, chives, eggs, and coconut milk. Mix it to form a ball.
- ❖ Drop the dough on to the already lined baking sheet with parchment paper. Flatten the dough and form a thick blanket of 1-inch in width.
- ❖ Cut them into 8 slices. Spread the cut slices to 2 inches apart.

❖ Bake for 20 minutes and garnish with more cheese and chives.

Chocolate Macaroons
Makes 10-15 macaroons
Calories 147, Protein 4g, Total Fat 6g, Carbohydrates 20g, Fiber 1g

Ingredients:
❖ 1 cup powdered sugar
❖ 1 tbsp. cocoa powder
❖ 1 cup ground almonds
❖ 2 medium egg whites
❖ 1 pinch salt
❖ ¼ cup powdered sugar (for the topping)

For the filling
❖ 1 oz. chocolate
❖ 2 tsp. of double cream (warm)

Directions:
❖ Preheat the oven to 365°F.
❖ In a large mixing bowl, sieve together your powdered sugar, cocoa powder, and almond meal.
❖ In a separate bowl, whisk together the egg whites until they form peaks. Add in a pinch of salt or crème of tartar while whisking the egg whites.
❖ Add the remaining powdered sugar and continue whisking until the whites are thick and glossy.

- ❖ Fold the icing sugar, cocoa powder, and almond mixture into the whites. Mix them all together with the help of a spatula using a cut and fold mixing technique. Do not over mix it.
- ❖ Fill a piping bag with a 1/3 inch nozzle, with the mixture.
- ❖ Line the parchment sheet onto the baking tray. Now gently pour out small blobs of the mixture through piping bag onto the sheet.
- ❖ Gently tap the baking sheet on the counter to let the mixture settle and any air bubbles to escape. Bake the macaroons for the next 15-20 minutes in the oven until the macaroons are firm and pop out of the parchment paper easily. You will notice the bubbly bottoms with the shiny, smooth top of your macaroons.
- ❖ Put your macaroons out in the air to allow them to cool completely while you are making the filling.
- ❖ Place a bowl over the saucepan of boiling water and add your grated chocolate chunks to melt.
- ❖ Once the chocolate is melted, pour in your cream and keep stirring until the mixture is blended completely, forming a ganache. Add a tsp. of butter for the gloss.
- ❖ Fill the filling onto the flat surface of the macaroon and sandwich it with another macaroon. Press gently.
- ❖ Repeat with the rest of the macaroons.

Peanut Butter Balls

Makes 15 balls
Calories 117.6, Protein 2.2g, Total Fat 6.6g,
Carbohydrates 13.7g, Fiber 0.5g

Ingredients:
- ❖ 1 ½ cups powdered sugar (sifted)
- ❖ ½ cup peanut butter creamy
- ❖ 4 tbsp. unsalted butter
- ❖ 1 semi sweetened dark chocolate bar

Directions:
- ❖ Mix the peanut butter with sugar and butter until all of it is incorporated.
- ❖ Once mixed, spoon out the mixture and roll it to form small balls.
- ❖ Place the balls on a lined baking sheet.
- ❖ Let the balls settle for the next 15 minutes until they dry.
- ❖ Crush or grate the chocolate bar into a bowl and melt it using a double boiler.
- ❖ Now dip the balls in the melted chocolate and coat them evenly.
- ❖ Remove the chocolate balls with the aid of a fork, dripping all the excess chocolate.
- ❖ Place them back on the waxed paper and let stand until it dries up.
- ❖ Store tightly in a covered and cool, dry place.

Gluten-free Peach Apple Crumble

Serves 4

Calories 204, Protein 2.7g, Total Fat 3.9g, Carbohydrates 52.1g, Fiber 4.6g

Ingredients:
- ❖ 1 ½ apple, peeled, cored and chopped
- ❖ 1 medium peach, peeled, pitted and chopped
- ❖ 2 1/3 tbsp. coconut sugar
- ❖ 2 1/3 tbsp. maple syrup
- ❖ 1 tsp. lemon juice
- ❖ ¾ tsp. vanilla extract
- ❖ ¾ tbsp. cornstarch
- ❖ ¾ tsp. ground cinnamon
- ❖ 2 1/3 tbsp. packed brown sugar
- ❖ 1/3 cup Gluten-free rolled oats
- ❖ ¼ cup almond flour
- ❖ 2 1/3 tbsp. unsalted butter, melted
- ❖ Sea salt and honey

Directions:
- ❖ Preheat the oven to 350°F.
- ❖ In a large bowl combine your fruits (apple and peaches), sugar, maple syrup, vanilla extract, lemon juice, and cinnamon powder.
- ❖ Now, add the corn starch and mix well to coat the fruits. Place in the bottom of a pie plate and set aside.

❖ In a separate mixing bowl, mix the remaining cinnamon, almond flour, butter, and brown sugar together.

❖ Place this crumble over the fruits and top it with the seasoning of sea salt.

❖ Cover the dish with tin foil and bake it for the next 20-25 minutes until the sugar has melted and the fruits have turned golden brown.

❖ Allow cooling before serving with vanilla ice cream scoop.

Poached Pears with Mascarpone

Serves 4

Calories 169, Protein 1g, Total Fat 7g, Carbohydrates 21g, Fiber 3g

Ingredients:
❖ 1 cup red wine
❖ 2 1/3 tbsp. maple syrup
❖ 1 tbsp. lemon juice
❖ ½ tsp. ground cinnamon
❖ 3 firm pears, peeled and cut in half
❖ 5 tbsp. of mascarpone cheese.

Directions:
❖ In a large saucepan, combine wine, lemon juice, maple syrup, and cinnamon. Bring this to a boil over medium-high heat.

- ❖ Reduce the heat to the medium and add the pears. Gently boil them for the next 10-12 minutes with the lid uncovered.
- ❖ Now turn the pears and boil for another 10 minutes until the pears are fork-tender.
- ❖ Remove the pears from the liquid and boil the liquid until it reduces to half.
- ❖ Serve ½ pear with the wine sauce topped with a tablespoon of mascarpone cheese.

Peanut Butter Mousse

Serves 4

Calories 258, Protein 10g, Total Fat 12g, Carbohydrates 31g, Fiber 2g

Ingredients:
- ❖ 12.3 oz. package of silken tofu
- ❖ 1/3 cup of creamy peanut butter
- ❖ Powdered sugar
- ❖ Toppings of your choice

Directions:
- ❖ Pour one 12.3 oz. package of silken tofu and 1/3 cup of creamy peanut butter and powdered sugar in a blender. Blend until smooth.
- ❖ Divide the mixture among glasses and cover with plastic wrap.
- ❖ Refrigerate the glasses for half an hour.

❖ Top it with the choices of your toppings (marshmallow, chopped peanuts or melted chocolate)

Easy Cheesecake
Makes 14 slices
Calories 229, Protein 11g, Total Fat 11g, Carbohydrates 24g, Fiber 2g

Ingredients:
❖ 9 low-fat gluten-free graham crackers (pulsed in a food processor)
❖ 3 - 4 tbsp. of melted unsalted butter.
❖ 4 packages (8 oz.) of cream cheese
❖ 1 ½ cup of coconut sugar
❖ 1 cup sour cream
❖ 2 large eggs at room temperature, and 3 egg whites separate
❖ 2 tbsp. multipurpose flour (gluten-free)
❖ 1 tsp. vanilla extract
❖ 1 tsp. Lemon or Orange Zest

Directions:
❖ Prepare your oven, preheat it to 350°F.
❖ Add your crumbled graham crackers to the food processor, and add melted butter with 2-3 tablespoons of water. Pulse well to moisten it.
❖ Coat the inner rim of the pan with cooking spray to grease the boundary.

- ❖ Place the crumbs at the bottom layer of the pan and press them gently with the aid of the glass bottom.
- ❖ Bake for 8 minutes until the color turns to brown. Let cool for 12 to 15 minutes.
- ❖ In a mixer, whip both your cream cheese and sugar until smooth.
- ❖ In a separate bowl, mix your eggs, flour, vanilla, and lemon zest. Mix until smooth.
- ❖ In another bowl, whisk your egg whites until they form stiff peaks. Add in a pinch of salt and continue whipping for another minute.
- ❖ Now pour the egg whites to the egg and flour batter and mix them using the cut and fold method.
- ❖ Pour the cheese mixture over the crust.
- ❖ Place the cheesecake in another large pan and add enough water to cover one-quarter of the way up the sides of the spring from the pan.
- ❖ Put the cake in the oven and bake until the cake is set, but the center still jiggles.
- ❖ Turn off the heat and let the cheesecake sit in the oven for another extra 20 minutes.
- ❖ Remove the cake from the oven and let it cool outside.
- ❖ Run a knife around the edge and let cool in the refrigerator for the next 4 hours or preferably overnight until the cake is set.
- ❖ Remove the springform pan and cut it into 14 equal slices.
- ❖ Serve as it is or have some caramel sauce drizzled on top.

Deep Dish Brownies

Makes 16 square brownies
Calories 158, Protein 2g, Total Fat 7g, Carbohydrates 23g, Fiber 0.5g

Ingredients:
* ❖ 3 tbsp. of unsalted butter (at room temperature)
* ❖ 2 tbsp. canola oil (or you can substitute it with butter)
* ❖ 4 oz. semi-sweet dark chocolate
* ❖ ¾ cup brown sugar
* ❖ ¼ cup coconut sugar
* ❖ 2 tsp. vanilla extract
* ❖ A pinch of salt
* ❖ 2 large eggs
* ❖ 1 tbsp. cold, instant coffee
* ❖ 2 ¼ cups of Dutch-process cocoa powder
* ❖ ¾ cup Multipurpose Flour (gluten-free)
* ❖ A pinch of baking soda

Directions:
* ❖ Preheat the oven to 325°F.
* ❖ Line a Pyrex glass baking dish with a parchment paper.
* ❖ Spray the pan to grease it completely.
* ❖ In a bowl, add butter, oil, and chocolate chunks and heat it either in a double boiler or microwave it periodically.
* ❖ Repeat the process every 30 seconds in the microwave until the chocolate is completely melted.

- ❖ Now in a separate bowl mix in your salt, white and brown sugar and transfer it into the chocolate mixture with a wooden spoon. At this point, you can add your vanilla extract.
- ❖ Now crack the eggs one by one, stirring continuously. Make sure the chocolate is warm and not hot so that it does not cook the eggs.
- ❖ Add your coffee to the mixture and mix well until the batter has reached a uniform consistency, and a glossy shine can be seen over the surface.
- ❖ Now add in the cocoa, flour, and baking soda and stir until well incorporated.
- ❖ Convert the batter into the baking dish and pop it into the oven until the crispy crust on the top is observed.
- ❖ Perform a toothpick test, if the toothpick comes out clean, you are good to go.
- ❖ Cool the brownies on the counter.
- ❖ Lift the brownies out of the dish and let them cool on the cooling rack.
- ❖ Peel off the parchment paper and cut the brownies in 3-inch squares.
- ❖ Serve them as it is or with a scoop of vanilla ice cream.

Broiled Banana

Serves 4

Calories 295, Protein 7g, Total Fat 8g, Carbohydrates 53g, Fiber 4g

Ingredients:
- ❖ 1 tbsp. of brown sugar
- ❖ ½ tsp. of cinnamon
- ❖ A pinch of salt
- ❖ 1 tbsp. of unsalted butter
- ❖ 2 Bananas (peeled and cut in half)
- ❖ Optional – add toppings of your choice (ice cream, frozen yogurt, almonds, fresh fruit)

Directions:
- ❖ Mix brown sugar, cinnamon powder, and a pinch of salt together.
- ❖ Brush 1 tbsp. melted butter on the sliced bananas and sprinkle with the cinnamon sugar.
- ❖ Wrap the bananas in foil and broil until golden. Top with frozen yogurt or ice cream, toasted almonds, and chopped chocolates.

Coconut Rice Pudding

Serves 4

Calories 150, Protein 2g, Total Fat 4g, Carbohydrates 27g, Fiber 1.5g

Ingredients:
- ❖ Cooking spray

- ❖ 1 ½ cups coconut water
- ❖ 1can (8 oz.) of lite coconut milk
- ❖ ¼ cup coconut sugar
- ❖ ½ tbsp. pure vanilla essence
- ❖ ¼ tsp. kosher salt
- ❖ ¾ cup brown rice, short-grained
- ❖ 1½ tbsp. of unsalted butter, cut into smaller pieces
- ❖ ½ tsp. lemon zest

Directions:
- ❖ With the help of a cooking spray, spray your slow cooker.
- ❖ Add coconut water, coconut milk, sugar, vanilla essence, and salt into the slow cooker.
- ❖ Put the cooker on the flame at low heat and keep stirring until the sugar is completely dissolved.
- ❖ Now pour in your rice in the same cooker and cook it on high setting for 4 hours.
- ❖ Uncover the slow cooker and stir well. Let it stand for 12 to 15 minutes.
- ❖ Transfer the mixture into a separate bowl and add your chunked butter to it.
- ❖ Once the butter is melted and well incorporated, let the dish settle until it gets warm.
- ❖ Stir in the lime zest and serve warm or chill until cold.
- ❖ Add toppings as desired.

References

Editors, R. D. (2017, December 19). Watch Out! These are the 4 Most Harmful Ingredients in Packaged Foods. Retrieved from https://www.thehealthy.com/nutrition/4-most-harmful-ingredients-in-packaged-foods/

Medicine, C. for V. (n.d.). Antimicrobial Resistance. Retrieved from https://www.fda.gov/animal-veterinary/safety-health/antimicrobial-resistance

Chang, K. (2012, September 4). Organic Food vs. Conventional Food. Retrieved from https://well.blogs.nytimes.com/2012/09/04/organic-food-vs-conventional-food

Ogden Publications, Inc. (n.d.). Good Calories, Bad Calories: What Makes Us Fat? Retrieved from https://www.motherearthnews.com/natural-health/good-calories-bad-calories-zmaz08onzgoe

Roseboro, K. (2019, January 31). Debunking 'Alternative Facts' About Pesticides and Organic Farming. Retrieved from https://www.ecowatch.com/pesticides-organic-farming-2292594453.html

Center for Food Safety and Applied Nutrition. (n.d.). Summary of Color Additives for Use in the United States. Retrieved from https://www.fda.gov/ForIndustry/ColorAdditives/C olorAdditiveInventories/ucm115641.html

Minal, J. (n.d.). Proposed FDA Rule To Ban Partially Hydrogenated (PHO) Oils . Retrieved from http://www.natuoil.com/wp-content/uploads/2014/02/2.-Proposed-Ban-of-Trans-Fats.pdf

Ucl. (2018, November 15). Brain and nervous system damaged by low-level exposure to pesticides. Retrieved from http://www.ucl.ac.uk/news/news-articles/1212/031212-Brain-and-nervous-system-damaged-by-rganophosphate-pesticides-MacKenzie-Ross

Gallagher, J. (2014, January 28). DDT: Pesticide linked to Alzheimer's. Retrieved from http://www.bbc.co.uk/news/health-25913568

Hutchison, C. (n.d.). ADHD From Allergy? Study Shows Benefit From Diet Changes. Retrieved from http://abcnews.go.com/Health/Allergies/adhd-food-allergy-case-restricting-diet/story?id=12832958

enter for Food Safety and Applied Nutrition. (n.d.). What You Need to Know about Food Allergies. Retrieved from https://www.fda.gov/Food/ResourcesForYou/Consu mers/ucm079311.htm

Bjarnadottir, A. (2019, January 3). 9 Popular Weight Loss Diets Reviewed. Retrieved from https://www.healthline.com/nutrition/9-weight-loss-diets-reviewed

7 Key Nutrients Vegetarians and Vegans Need to Watch. (2010, July 20). Retrieved from https://www.sparkpeople.com/resource/nutrition_art icles.asp?id=1530

Harvard Health Publishing. (n.d.). Becoming a vegetarian. Retrieved from https://www.health.harvard.edu/staying-healthy/becoming-a-vegetarian

Which Digestive Organ Absorbs Nutrients? | Healthfully. (n.d.). Retrieved from https://www.livestrong.com/article/436603-in-which-digestive-organ-are-nutrients-absorbed/

Hyman, M. (n.d.). How Good Gut Health Can Boost Your Immune System. Retrieved from https://www.ecowatch.com/how-good-gut-health-can-boost-your-immune-system-1882013643.html

s3rdopinion. (2017, March 1). Gut & Digestive... Retrieved from https://3rdopinion.us/functional-medicine/gut-digestive-health/

Dănuț, Î. (2017, February 5). Why and How Your State of Mind Affects Your Gut, and Vice Versa! Retrieved from https://www.sociedelic.com/why-and-how-your-state-of-mind-affects-your-gut-and-vice-versa/

Erik, Griffiths, D., Nadia, Nadia, Catherine, Raivon, … Grimes, G. (2019, September 17). How to Use Apple Cider Vinegar to Improve Digestion. Retrieved from https://bodyunburdened.com/use-apple-cider-vinegar-improve-digestion/

Link, R. (2019, August 13). This 'Immortal Health Elixir' Protects Your Gut & Fights Food Poisoning Pathogens (and More!). Retrieved from https://draxe.com/7-reasons-drink-kombucha-everyday/

Galland, J. (2016, August 31). A Gut-Healthy Fruit That Fights Inflammation (That You Can Eat All Year Round). Retrieved from https://www.mindbodygreen.com/0-26402/a-guthealthy-fruit-that-fights-inflammation-that-you-can-eat-all-year-round.html

Lewin, J. (1970, May 25). What does organic mean? Retrieved from https://www.bbcgoodfood.com/howto/guide/organic